EMERGENCY MEDICINE

MEDICAL SCHOOL CRASH COURSE

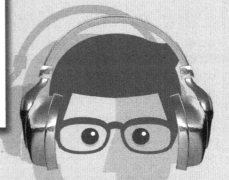

HIGH-YIELD CONTENT REVIEW

Q&A AND "KEY TAKEAWAYS"

TOP 100 TEST QUESTIONS

FOLLOW-ALONG PDF MANUAL

audio learn™

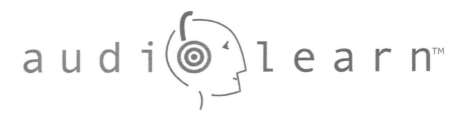

EMERGENCY MEDICINE

Medical School Crash Course[TM]

www.AudioLearn.com

Table of Contents

Preface

Emergency medicine involves the care of many different types of patients, some of whom are critically-ill, while others only have illnesses requiring observation and the basics of management. This course is intended to cover the basics of emergency medicine presentations as well as the emergency medicine workup techniques necessary to identify serious medical problems. The care of these patients and their disposition are also part of this course.

The first aspect in the care of the critically-ill, injured, or compromised patient is the establishment of an airway, which is the first topic covered in the first chapter of this course. The care of these individuals requires an evaluation of the individual's airway patency and the ability of the patient to take a spontaneous breath. For either problem, the patient will need an artificial airway. This first chapter is about the evaluation and practice of airway management in the patient who requires oxygenation.

The second chapter of the course is a discussion of the phenomenon of "shock". The definition of shock is more complex that just the finding of low blood pressure. There are a wide variety of systemic complications that occur because of shock, the most serious of which is end-organ failure of the major organs, such as the kidneys and liver. This chapter covers two of the more common types of shock seen in emergency medicine, including cardiogenic shock and distributive shock.

Cardiac resuscitation is the topic of the third chapter of the course. Cardiac resuscitation is the emergency medical response to a cardiac arrest situation, which, in turn, usually results from a severe myocardial infarction with a severe arrhythmia, although things like a pulmonary embolism, ventricular wall rupture, low potassium levels, heavy exercise, and major blood loss can cause a cardiac arrest. This chapter will discuss the phenomenon of the cardiac arrest as well as the emergency medical response to this type of catastrophic event.

One of the more common things an emergency medicine physician will have to deal with is the febrile patient, which is the topic of discussion in the fourth chapter of the course. Most patients with fever will have some type of infection that needs to be discovered and managed. Less commonly, the cause of fever will be unrelated to an infection. This chapter focuses on the febrile patient, including the workup of fever, the diagnosis of fever, and the treatment of fever and febrile illnesses.

Chest pain is the topic of chapter five in this course. Chest pain in the adult emergency department patient can be serious or benign but always need to be worked up by the emergency room physician in order to identify which types of chest pain need further intervention and which can simply be monitored. This chapter discusses both the phenomenon of chest pain and the possible things that can cause this important symptom.

The sixth chapter in the course covers the emergency medicine topic of head trauma. The head trauma patient may have a concussion or other minor injury and they may have either an open head injury (penetrating) or a closed head injury (blunt trauma). Injuries can also be very severe, resulting in severe brain contusions and intracerebral bleeding that can be life-threatening if not treated soon and aggressively.

The seventh chapter in the course involves a thorough discussion of eye injuries. Injury is the most common reason for eye-related emergency department (ED) visits. The incidence of eye injuries requiring emergency department medical attention in the US is estimated to be between 500 and 1000 patients per 100,000 population. This chapter will cover some of the more common eye injuries seen in emergency medicine along with the treatment of these diseases.

The eighth chapter of the course involves the impact of chest trauma in an emergency department patient. Chest trauma can occur secondary to many different things, including penetrating injuries, falls, and motor vehicle accidents. The different things that can cause chest trauma can affect the heart or the lungs, leading to cardiorespiratory compromise. This chapter will cover both blunt traumatic injuries of the chest and penetrating injuries of the chest and their implications.

The ninth chapter in the course is a thorough discussion of abdominal trauma and its manifestations. Because there are many vital organs in the abdomen and pelvis, trauma to these areas is hardly ever benign. The patient with abdominal trauma can have damage to any of the solid organs in the abdomen or any part of the abdominal viscus. Infections tend to be common late manifestations of abdominal trauma as the viscus of the abdomen carries billions of microorganisms—some of them pathogenic. The purpose of this chapter is to discuss the basics of abdominal trauma and its management.

The tenth chapter in this course is devoted to discussing the evaluation and management of the acute abdomen and the related phenomenon of pelvic pain. These are common problems in emergency medicine and require a systematic approach that attempts to distinguish between a non-operative condition and those that require surgical intervention. The definition of the "acute abdomen" is one that ultimately needs surgery to treat the patient's abdominal or pelvic complaints.

The major topic discussed in chapter eleven is the management of patients with multiple trauma. It is not uncommon for the emergency room physician to encounter a patient who has the confounding problem of having multiple areas of trauma secondary to a motor vehicle accident, a fall, or other serious injury. These patients need to be managed in a manner that addresses the more serious problems first, followed by a systematic assessment and management of the less serious injuries.

The emergency care of lacerations and other wounds is the subject of the twelfth chapter in the course. The treatment of skin wounds includes mainly the treatment of lacerations, abrasions, and puncture wounds—each of which are treated slightly differently. These are extremely common skin problems affecting nearly everyone at some point in their lives. The goal of the emergency medical physician or dermatologist is to determine what kind of wound the patient has and to use the proper protocols for each of these skin wounds. The focus of this chapter is on the management of wounds and the specific techniques used in emergency laceration repair.

Chapter 13 of the course involves the care and management of psychiatric emergencies. A psychiatric emergency can be defined as any situation in which the healthcare provider confronts a situation in which the patient cannot stop acting on compulsions to harm themselves or another person. The patient may present with full awareness of the impact of their desired behavior but more often than not, they present with a lack of judgment and insight into what might happen should they follow through on their compulsion.

The study of toxicology in the emergency department is the topic of the fourteenth chapter of the book. This involves both the study of toxic medications that are not normally toxic under typical situations but become toxic in high doses and a discussion of things that are always toxic to the body. There are some things that are toxic to the kidneys, toxic to the heart, toxic to the lungs, toxic to a growing fetus, or toxic to the ears. Each of these is discussed in this chapter.

Chapter 1: Airway Management

The first aspect in the care of the critically-ill, injured, or compromised patient is the establishment of an airway. This requires an evaluation of the individual's airway patency and the ability of the patient to take a spontaneous breath. For either problem, the patient will need an artificial airway. This chapter is about the evaluation and practice of airway management in the patient who requires oxygenation.

Airway Basics

The first task of the emergency medicine physician or healthcare provider is to assess the patient's airway. This is done even before evaluating their spontaneous breathing capabilities. The first thing the provider must do is perform a jaw thrust maneuver in order open the airway. This can be done on any patient, even those suspected of having a cervical spine injury. If the airway is *patent*, the patient may then spontaneously breathe.

There are several major reasons to intubate the patient. These include the following:

- Lack of airway patency

- Need for positive pressure ventilation (such as hypercarbia or hypoxic situations)

- Shock or other cardiovascular compromise

- Head injury, seizures, or other neurologic problems affecting respirations

- Inhalation injury to the airways or lungs

- Possibility of clinical deterioration

Intubation is just one step in oxygenating the patient and isn't always required. Patients die not from a lack of intubation but from a lack of adequate degree of oxygenation, which can be provided in any number of ways. Nevertheless, the gold standard, however, for providing a secure airway is endotracheal intubation.

Figure 1 shows endotracheal intubation:

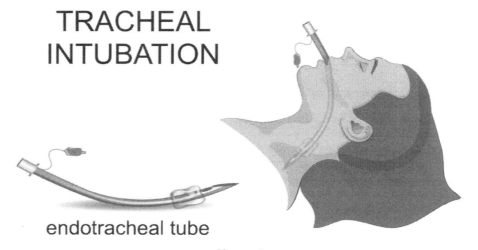

TRACHEAL INTUBATION

endotracheal tube

Figure 1

In assessing the airway, it is necessary first to assess its patency. If the jaw-thrust maneuver doesn't provide for spontaneous respirations, the airway can be evaluated for a foreign body. Suctioning, if available, should be done along with continuous maintenance of a good anatomical position for the best patency.

The oral airway device may be adequate for the patient who is spontaneously breathing or in cases where a bag-valve mask is necessary. This should be used in the unconscious patient only as it can precipitate the gag reflex and may induce vomiting in the conscious patient. It can be inserted upside down and then twisted into position after it has been advanced or a tongue blade can be used to hold the tongue down while putting the airway in place.

Another option is a nasopharyngeal airway. These are placed directly through the nostril and into the upper pharynx, where it reaches as far down as the hypopharynx. They can cause epistaxis but are more easily tolerated in a conscious patient. They are simply lubricated and placed into the nostril. It is made from soft, flexible rubber-like material and KY is generally the lubricant of choice for this airway.

Bag Valve Mask

Bag-valve mask ventilation is done before obtaining the definitive, protected airway. It can be used in a partially conscious patient who is underventilated. Ideally, it is a two-person job, with one person holding the valve in place and the other person squeezing the bag. This is a self-inflating bag that acts like an oxygen reservoir that is linked to a non-rebreathing exhalation valve or NRV. The valve is clear so as to evaluate the patient continuously for vomiting. It should deliver about 800 ml of oxygen per breath.

Figure 2 shows what a bag-valve mask looks like:

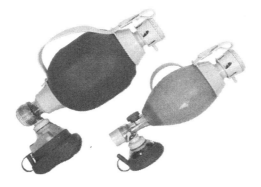

Figure 2

The mask should be the smallest mask to fit over the nose and mouth because this provides the least dead air space and will be easier to handle. The mask should not be forced hard on the face as it can cause misalignment of the airway. It simply needs to create a tight seal around the nose and mouth. Ventilations should have a slow inspiratory phase at 1-2 seconds with a low airway pressure to minimize inflation of the stomach with air.

The mainstay of BVM (bag-valve mask) ventilation is to have a good seal and to deliver an adequate volume per breath. The goal is to ventilate the patient until a definitive airway can be established.

Things like facial hair and missing teeth can make this a difficult task. Facial trauma has also been implicated in casing problems with BMV ventilation. When one person is doing this job, the non-dominant hand should be in a C-shape (holding the mask over the mouth and nose), while the dominant hand squeezes the bag. Dentures should be left in place in order to provide an adequate seal.

Endotracheal Intubation

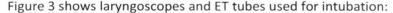

The definitive airway is the cuffed endotracheal tube that both protects the airway from aspiration and provides positive-pressure ventilation. The cuff is placed below the glottis in the trachea so that both lungs can be equally ventilated. It is often the most lifesaving thing that can be done to ventilate the patient. Patients with any of the issues listed above, including the potential for deterioration should be considered for endotracheal intubation, particularly if they need transportation to definitive care and intubation would be difficult during transport.

There are a number of ETT (endotracheal tube) sizes that are usually labeled by the millimeters of internal diameter. The typical ET tube size for an adult is 7 mm internal diameter. The largest size should be selected to minimize airway resistance but it shouldn't be so big as to cause trauma to the trachea. A balloon on the end has air inserted into it at about 5-10 ml per balloon tip. Intubation is done with a semi-rigid stylet in difficult cases with the tip of the stylet ending about 1-2 cm before the end of the ETT tube. It cannot be extended past the tip of the ET tube.

The laryngoscope is a metallic, rigid instrument that is necessary for intubating the trachea because visualization of the vocal cords is necessary. There are two main types of blades used in the US. The Macintosh blade is a curved blade where the tip is inserted into the vallecular space. The straight laryngoscope is the Miller blade that lifts the epiglottis in order to expose the vocal cords. They come in large, medium, and small sizes.

Figure 3 shows laryngoscopes and ET tubes used for intubation:

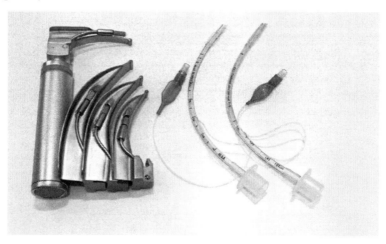

Figure 3

Preoxygenation is necessary before intubation in order to have a lung reserve of oxygen. This involves giving 100 percent oxygen by a non-rebreather mask or bag-valve mask for a couple of minutes before intubation. This will prolong the time before desaturation occurs during the intubation process, which may take a while if the intubation is difficult. Older adults, obese patients, and children particularly need preoxygenation as they desaturate faster and have more problems with a poor oxygen reserve.

In preoxygenating with a bag-valve mask, the bag should contain 100 percent O2 and should be squeezed every five seconds with enough air to cause chest rising. Too forcible ventilations can cause gastric distention and possible vomiting. Ventilation should be about 10-12 breaths per minute with a smaller volume used when CPR is being performed. The BMV device cannot be used in facial trauma that is so severe as to cause upper airway obstruction or a lack of seal of the mask. A surgical airway must be used in these cases.

Patients should be assessed for the possibility of a difficult airway before attempting the intubation. The mnemonic "LEMON" is used to assess the intubation difficulty. The mnemonic "LEMON" stands for this:

- **L**—Look for obesity, head and neck problems, facial hair, poor teeth, high arched palate, obesity or a short, thick neck.

- **E**—Evaluate the 3-3-2 rule, which is mouth opening of at least three fingerbreadths, a hyomental distance of at least three fingerbreadths, and the thyrohyoid distance of at least 2 fingerbreadths.

- **M**—Mallampati classification. This involves asking the patient to open their mouth. The easiest airway includes those where all structures can be seen when the patient opens their mouth.

- **O**—this involves any type of obstruction to intubation, including swelling, facial trauma, or excessive soft tissue.

- **N**—This involves an evaluation for neck mobility. This may not be possible in situations where the patient is in a neck brace.

Rapid Sequence Intubation

Rapid sequence intubation or RSI involves a method of doing an intubation in a patient that might carry an aspiration risk. It involves two main components: induction first and then paralysis. The first part (induction) involves creating an unresponsive state in the patient—usually with etomidate or propofol. This is followed by paralyzing the patient with succinylcholine or vecuronium. The technique of RSI improves the success rate of the intubation process, decreases the aspiration risk, and offers better cervical spine control.

The downside and risks of doing the RSI include a longer time of intubation, the development of a "crash airway" in which intubation is essential, and adverse effects from the drug. Patients who are in cardiac arrest are not candidates nor do they need RSI. The patient should be preoxygenated and evaluated while receiving BVM ventilation with 100 percent O2 before paralytics are given.

The patient should be adequately positioned before intubating. This includes tilting the head (unless there is possible spine trauma), jaw-thrust maneuver, and applying upward/backward pressure on the thyroid cartilage in order to allow for better positioning of the vocal cords. The jaw-thrust maneuver involves pushing the jaw forward without bending back the neck in suspected spine conditions.

It should be noted that paralysis may take a while after the paralytic agent is given. This means that the provider should monitor the patient for muscle fasciculations. When these stop, the patient should be adequately paralyzed and the ETT can be placed. The larynx is visualized with the laryngoscope after pushing the tongue to one side. The dominant hand is used to insert the ETT through the vocal cords while having the nondominant hand using the laryngoscope to pull tissues out of the way. The teeth should not be used for leverage when the tube is being placed as this can break off teeth.

The tip of the tube should be visualized along with the cords so that the tube is actually seen passing the cords. It should be advanced so the tip of the ETT is in the trachea and the cuff can be inflated. It is only then that positive pressure ventilations can be established. The lungs should be auscultated bilaterally to make sure the breath sounds are equal and end-tidal CO_2 should be measured as the most accurate way of determining ET tube placement. A chest x-ray can be done but this isn't as good a way of determining the ETT placement as is the end-tidal CO_2 level.

The tube's balloon cuff needs about 5-10 cc of air and the tube should be secured with tape to the patient's face. The abdomen should be auscultated to make sure that the tube has not been placed in the esophagus. Pulse oximetry can also be helpful in determining the adequacy of ETT placement. The chest x-ray is a good way of determining the depth of the tube's tip. It can also tell if there is a pneumothorax or other lung complication of positive pressure ventilation. Arterial blood gases can be another tool for detecting an adequate ventilation status.

Laryngeal Mask Airway

Both the Combitube Laryngeal Mask Airway (LMA) and the King Laryngeal Tube (LT) are commonly used by prehospital personnel to provide oxygen to the patient if an ETT cannot be placed. It works by occluding the esophagus and blindly intubating the trachea preferentially. It allows for a protected airway and positive pressure ventilation.

The LMA is a device with a cuff that is large enough to occlude the esophagus. It has special usefulness when the vocal cords can't be visualized in a cervical spine injured patient. It isn't as protective of the airway as an ETT so it is desirable to switch to an ET tube intubation as soon as it is feasible. The most common use of this device is in trauma patients who can't be bagged with the BVM and can't easily be intubated. It tends to be more reliable that BVM so is an option in the care of the patient needing a good ventilation source. The LMA devices come in different sizes with the size clearly marked on the tube.

Figure 4 shows what a laryngeal mask airway looks like:

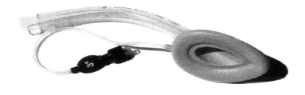

Figure 4

To do an LMA insertion, the first step is to inflate the cuff to make sure it doesn't leak. It should then be deflated so it will easy pass over the tongue and behind the epiglottis. A water-soluble lubricant can help the passage of the tube. The patient should be in the sniffing position unless they have a suspected cervical spine injury. The tube should be inserted until resistance is noted. Then the cuff should be inflated just enough to obtain a seal. A ventilator bag should then be attached and the patient's breath sounds should be auscultated for ventilations. End-tidal CO2 measurement is the preferable way of determining accurate placement of the LMA. Remember that vomiting and aspiration are possible in an alert patient.

Surgical Airway

If attempts at oral intubation has failed or there is a great deal of facial trauma, a surgical airway may be necessary in the form of a surgical cricothyroidotomy. This may be necessary, even in the field. There are kits that can be opened and used for this purpose. Patients with clenched teeth, massive pharyngeal hemorrhage, masseter muscle spasm, laryngospasm, structural oropharyngeal problems, or airway obstruction should have a surgical airway. The kids come with a tracheostomy tube and there are different sizes of tubes—all of which are cuffed. Select a tube that is about 75 percent of the diameter of the trachea.

Figure 5 shows where a surgical airway is performed:

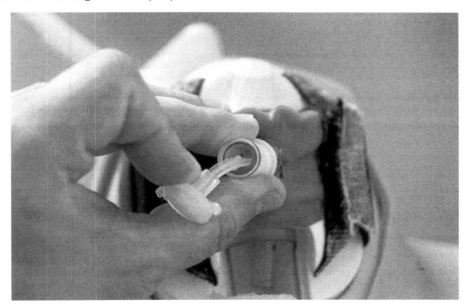

Figure 5

The incision should be vertical and about 1.5 cm over the cricothyroid membrane with a secondary horizontal cut through the membrane itself. Once the membrane has been breached, the cricoid cartilage is hooked with a tracheal hook. Then the membrane is dilated using traction. A cuffed size 4 tracheostomy tube or a cuffed size 6.0 ETT tube should be introduced into the trachea. Sometimes, an elastic bougie is placed into the trachea with the tube passed over that. The cuff can then be inflated in the trachea with the usual measurements of end-tidal CO2 levels done to make sure the tube is in proper position. The tube can finally be sutured in place.

Extubation of the Intubated Patient

At some point, the patient needs to be extubated. The first step in doing this is deflating the balloon so there is confirmed air leak around the ETT. If this isn't the case, there can be stridor and upper airway obstruction secondary to edema of the trachea. Decadron can be given IV before Extubation (at around four hours pre-extubation and continued every six hours for 3-4 doses) in order to help prevent inflammation and edema. The patient should have nothing orally before intubation as there can be aspiration if the patient needs to be re-intubated. There should be confirmation of alertness and spontaneous breathing with good oxygenation demonstrated. Epinephrine nebulizer therapy should be available to reduce stridor. Suction should happen first and then removal of the ETT, with careful following of the patient's respiratory status.

Key Takeaways

- The airway is the first thing that needs assessment in caring for the critically-ill or traumatized patient.

- The endotracheal tube is the gold standard for providing a secure airway in a critically-ill patient.

- The BVM is generally a two-person job but is the best way to preoxygenate a patient before intubating.

- The LMA can be used on cervical spine patients and when an ETT is not possible.

- If attempts at an oral airway are not successful, a surgical airway is the treatment of choice.

Quiz

1. In evaluating the airway in a compromised patient, what is the first step necessary to evaluate the patency of the airway?

   a. Listen for breath sounds

   b. Perform the jaw thrust maneuver

   c. Tip the neck back and open the mouth

   d. Sweep the mouth for foreign bodies

Answer: b. The jaw-thrust maneuver will be done in evaluating the patency of the airway. It will open the air passage and will allow for spontaneous respirations if they are going to occur.

2. There are many indications for intubation. What is not necessarily a requirement for intubation?

   a. Lack of patent airway

   b. Hypercarbia and need for positive pressure ventilation

   c. Shock

   d. Agitation

Answer: d. The main reasons for intubation include all of the above except for agitation.

3. For what reason should an oral airway only be used in an unconscious patient?

    a. It can push the tongue into the path of the airway in a conscious patient.

    b. This type of airway intervention is not necessary in a conscious patient.

    c. Conscious patients will have an induction of vomiting and gagging with oral airways.

    d. Conscious patients often spit out oral airways.

Answer: c. An oral airway should be avoided in a conscious patient because conscious patients will have a gag reflex and possible vomiting when an oral airway is used.

4. For which type of patient is preoxygenation before intubation indicated because of poor oxygen reserves?

    a. Elderly patients

    b. Children

    c. Obese patients

    d. All of the above

Answer: d. All of these types of patients need preoxygenation as they have a poor oxygen reserve compared to healthy patients of an adult age.

5. When preoxygenating a patient, what is the approximate rate at which ventilations should be given?

    a. 5-6 ventilations per minute

    b. 6-8 ventilations per minute

    c. 8-10 ventilations per minute

    d. 10-12 ventilations per minute

Answer: d. A total of about 10-12 ventilations per minute should be given in order to preoxygenate the patient before intubation.

6. Which is the most effective way of preoxygenating a patient for intubation?

    a. 100 percent O2 by bag-valve mask

    b. 4 liters of oxygen by mask

    c. 100 percent O2 by nonrebreather mask

    d. 2 liters oxygen by nasal cannula

Answer: a. The most effective way of preoxygenating a patient for intubation is to use a bag-valve mask and to provide 100 percent oxygen. The other ways are less effective at preoxygenating the patient.

7. What is considered a main advantage of doing RSI versus regular endotracheal intubation?

    a. It can be used on patients with facial trauma

    b. It is faster than a regular intubation

    c. It relatively protects the patient from aspiration

    d. It is safer than regular intubation in children

Answer: c. RSI allows for intubation in patients who have a risk for aspiration and can be done in patients who were conscious or semi-conscious at the time of their intubation as it renders the patient unconscious and paralyzed.

8. Which of the following patients should not have the RSI procedure when intubating them?

    a. The cervical spine-injured patient

    b. The head trauma patient

    c. The septic patient

    d. The cardiac arrest patient

Answer: d. The patient with a cardiac arrest does not need and should not have RSI. They can adequately be ventilated with a regular intubation procedure.

9. What is the major downside of doing the RSI procedure?

    a. It can create a "crash airway" situation

    b. It cannot be done on the semi-conscious patient

    c. It cannot be done on the cervical spine-injured patient

    d. It requires an IV access

Answer: a. The main downsides of the RSI technique is that it takes longer than a regular intubation, there are side effects from the medications, and it can create a "crash airway" situation.

10. When extubating a patient, what can be given before the procedure in order to make sure the patient has a decreased chance of tracheal edema?

    a. Epinephrine IV

    b. Decadron IV

    c. Epinephrine nebulizer

    d. Albuterol nebulizer

Answer: b. Decadron can be given intravenously before extubation in order to prevent tracheal edema after removing the tube.

Chapter 2: Shock

The definition of shock is more complex that just the phenomenon of low blood pressure. There are a wide variety of systemic complications that occur because of shock, the most serious of which is end-organ failure of the major organs, such as the kidneys and liver. This chapter will cover two of the more common types of shock seen in emergency medicine, including cardiogenic shock and distributive shock.

Cardiogenic Shock

The most basic definition of cardiogenic shock is a low cardiac output with tissue hypoxia of the peripheral tissues in the presence of an essentially normal intravascular volume. This is the most common cause of death in cases of acute myocardial infarction with a mortality rate that approaches 90 percent unless the patient is aggressively managed.

Figure 6 describes the organs affected by cardiogenic shock:

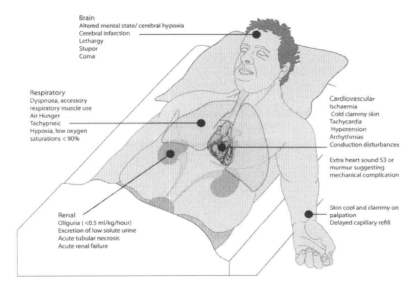

Figure 6

Shock as a diagnosis may sometimes be made clinically by noting the following findings on clinical examination:

- Decreased blood pressure (below 90 systolic)

- No evidence of dehydration and hypovolemia

- Evidence f tissue hypoperfusion (cyanosis, oliguria, change in mental status, and cold extremities)

- Central or peripheral cyanosis

- Rapid and sometimes irregular pulse

- Faint peripheral pulses

- Muffled heart sounds on auscultation

Imaging studies that should be performed include an echocardiogram, which will show wall motion abnormalities in an acute MI, valvular disease (such as a ruptured mitral valve papillary muscle), or marked cardiomegaly. A chest x-ray can be done to show other causes of shock, such as pneumo-mediastinum, tension pneumothorax, or an aortic dissection. If the patient is in the acute stages of a suspected myocardial infarction, a coronary angioplasty is indicated so as to perform an emergency angioplasty or other revascularization procedure before there is maximal tissue necrosis.

Other tests and workup include an electrocardiogram to evaluate the patient for an acute MI, keeping in mind that a normal ECG may still be present in the face of a myocardial infarction. All patients with shock should have a Swan-Ganz catheter placed to further delineate their fluid status and central venous pressures. This will help in the diagnosis of pump failure and in managing their overall fluid status.

Swan-Ganz Catheter Utilization

The Swan-Ganz catheter is helpful in caring for the shock patient as well as in diagnosing the cause of certain cardiac conditions. It is also referred to as a pulmonary artery catheter or "right-heart catheter" because it measures the pressures in the pulmonary artery. It is widely used in critical care medicine.

Indications for a Swan-Ganz or PAC catheter include its use diagnostically in suspected acute right heart syndrome, suspected coronary arterial disease, and for new-onset left heart failure. It can be used therapeutically for aspiration of an air embolus in the pulmonary vasculature.

It is probably not acceptable to use this device during low-risk CAD cases, in the management of patients having a coronary angiogram, or in cases of arrhythmia, such as heart block or atrial flutter. It is not appropriate for patients undergoing low-risk coronary artery surgery, in patients with mitral disease or aortic valve disease, or in patients with symptomatic prosthetic valve disease.

The PAC in generally inserted via a major vein (which can be the femoral vein, subclavian vein, or jugular vein) by means of an introducer sheath. The Shortest path to the heart is the right internal jugular vein but the left subclavian vein doesn't require passing the catheter through a sharp angle. The femoral vein route can be more difficult and has an access point greater than the other two. These are the best sites when hemorrhage is suspected.

Sterile technique must be adhered to with a large draped area because the PAC is about 150 cm in total length. The Trendelenburg position is used for internal jugular or subclavian techniques. After insertion, the patient is placed upright in order to pass the catheter. The balloon function should be assessed before insertion. The catheter should be flushed with IV fluid with air bubbles removed before insertion and all lumens should be connected to stopcocks. It should be covered with a sterile sheath for sterile manipulation of the catheter.

The catheter has a preformed curve that helps it pass easier into the pulmonary artery (PA). The curve should be directed so that the tip can easily slide into the PA. After 20 cm (upper vein) or 30 cm (femoral vein) have been passed into the body, the balloon should be inflated slowly up to 1.5 ml volume. It should always be inflated before advancing and deflated before withdrawing. Monitoring of the pressures should happen while advancing the catheter.

Eventually the PA is entered and the PCWP can be measured (pulmonary capillary wedge pressure). Determine the volume of air that was introduced into the balloon before removing the sterile field and taping the catheter down. In general, the PCWP is the same as the PA diastolic pressure, which is a measurement of left ventricular filling pressure. A chest x-ray should be obtained to check for a pneumothorax and other complications (and to assess the placement of the catheter).

Things that can be measured with the PAC include the systemic vascular resistance, the pulmonary vascular resistance, the cardiac output, the oxygen delivery to the heart, the oxygen consumption, the arterial oxygen content, the venous oxygen content, the oxygen extraction ratio, the intrapulmonary shunt, and the blood pressures in the aorta, left ventricle, pulmonary artery, and left atrium.

When the PCWP is determined, it is the pressure found when the balloon occludes the pulmonary vasculature so that the balloon stops antegrade blood flow and allows an uninterrupted column of blood to exist between the catheter tip and the LA. This provides an accurate measurement of the left ventricular filling pressure.

Management of Cardiogenic Shock

The phenomenon of cardiogenic shock is an emergency situation, requiring aggressive management. If the patient does not have pulmonary edema, they should have fluid resuscitation to improve hypotension. There are a number of helpful drugs (to be discussed) that are given intravenously. An ICU admission is essential and the two major emphases are to restore coronary blood flow and to correct the most common electrolyte/acid-base problems, which are low potassium levels, low magnesium levels, and acidosis.

Invasive things that should be done include placing a central line, placing an arterial line (to continually monitor the blood pressure and provide good venous access, and placing an intra-aortic balloon pump in order to support the heart before revascularization.

There are a number of drugs used in the management of these patients. These include aspirin (as an antiplatelet drug), heparin (to prevent clot formation), inotropic or vasopressor drugs (to maintain tissue perfusion), and diuretics (to manage pulmonary edema and peripheral edema).

The vasopressor of choice is dopamine because it increases cardiac contractility. It is started at 5-10 mcg/kg/min intravenously, with increases in dose titrated to the blood pressure. Doses may reach 20 mcg/kg/min, which is the maximum recommended dose. It may increase the oxygen demand on the heart. If maximal doses are given, then norepinephrine at 0.5 mcg/kg/min is given until the MAP (mean arterial pressure) is at least 60 mm Hg. The maximum dose of norepinephrine is 3.3 mcg/kg/min.

If the blood pressure is greater than 80 mg Hg systolic, dobutamine may be used and has the advantage of not increasing the myocardial oxygen demand as much. It can lead to unwanted tachycardia, however.

Two phosphodiesterase inhibitors can be used as they are inotropic and cause vasodilation. These include milrinone and Inamrinone (amrinone). They have long half-lives but may need a vasopressor alongside their use as they can lower the systemic blood pressure.

The treatment of choice in cardiogenic shock is either a percutaneous coronary intervention (PCI) or the CABG procedure. PCI needs to happen within 90 minutes of arrival to the ED but it can help if done within 12 hours after admission. If these two techniques are not available, thrombolytic therapy is indicated as a second-line therapy.

It should be remembered that the treatment of shock should happen as soon as possible in order to avoid irreversible end-organ damage. Blood pressure support, respiratory support, and cardiac output all need to be addressed as well as managing the underlying cause of the problem. These are critically-ill patients that need ICU admission and restoration of coronary artery perfusion.

The medical treatments given to patients with ACS (acute coronary syndrome) and shock should include aspirin, heparin, dopamine, dobutamine, epinephrine, and norepinephrine. The goal for vasopressors is to have a MAP of at least 60 mm Hg for adequate tissue perfusion. Clopidogrel should be started after the angiography and, if a CABG is warranted, it should be given after that procedure. Glycoprotein IIb/IIIa blockers seem to be helpful in caring for NSTEMI cases and will reduce the risk of another MI.

While thrombolytic therapy is considered a second-line agent for cardiogenic shock. It reduces the likelihood of developing cardiogenic shock when it doesn't exist at the time of treatment but doesn't improve mortality rates after cardiogenic shock has already begun with a mortality rate of about 70 percent when thrombolytics are used.

The intra-aortic balloon pump or IABP can help the patient with cardiogenic shock after other treatments fail. The IABP will reduce the LV afterload and will help augment the diastolic coronary perfusion pressure. It is helpful in the initial stages but is not a long-term therapy. It helps people who are scheduled for some type of revascularization procedure. It has a 30 percent complication rate, including hemolysis, infection, embolism, or local vascular problems. It works better before shock has developed.

Left ventricular assist devices or LVADs can support the heart after acute occlusion of the coronary arteries and causes reduction of the left ventricular preload, increasing the regional myocardial blood flow (which improves heart function). It maintains the aortic pressure and cardiac output on a temporary basis. These can be implanted and used in patients awaiting a heart transplant.

As mentioned, the definitive treatment for cardiogenic shock is some type of revascularization procedure, such as a PTCA (percutaneous transluminal coronary angioplasty). This can provide for adequate blood flow in up to 90 percent of cases (versus 60 percent of cases after thrombolytic therapy). The time from admission to procedure needs to be as short as possible in order to have the best outcome.

Patients who have cardiogenic shock often have critical mainstem arterial disease or three-vessel disease, sometimes so severe that a percutaneous coronary intervention can't be performed. These patients are candidates for CABG, which can restore arterial blood flow to the heart. Surgery has a higher mortality rate than a PCI procedure so it shouldn't be considered a first-line treatment, even though it is more successful than medical therapy alone. The one-year survival rate for the CABG procedure in cardiogenic shock patients is about 47 percent versus 34 percent in people who were not revascularized.

Distributive Shock

Distributive shock happens because of excessive vasodilation of the vasculature, with septic shock being the most common type of this kind of shock. The other causes of distributive shock include anaphylactic shock, neurogenic shock (in a spinal cord injury), reaction to drugs or toxins, heavy metal toxicity, shock secondary to an inflammatory response (such as pancreatitis and burns), toxic shock syndrome, liver failure, and adrenal crisis (from a lack of steroid hormones).

Distributive shock is just one type of the four different types of shock, including cardiogenic shock (from heart pump failure), hypovolemic shock (from intravascular volume loss), or obstructive shock (a blockage of the circulation of the blood).

SIRS can be caused by any of the following: burns, infections, traumatic injuries, pancreatitis, surgery, and severe liver failure. The diagnosis of shock secondary to "systemic inflammatory response" or SIRS is made by having at least 2 out of 4 separate criteria, including:

- Fever of at least 100 degrees Fahrenheit or hypothermia of less than 96.8 degrees Fahrenheit.

- Heart rate in excess of 90 BPM.

- Respirations of greater than 20 breaths per minute or a PaCO2 of less than 32 mmHg.

- WBC count of less than 4000 cells per microliter or greater than 12,000 cells per microliter (or more than 10 percent bands in the peripheral smear).

In distributive shock, the arteries are dilated so that there is a low blood pressure and a lack of adequate tissue perfusion. The normal responses of the smooth muscles of the arteries don't happen and the patient has an increased tissue ischemia with increased serum lactate levels. The blood pressure decreases and there is an increase in capillary refill. The cardiac output is increased in an attempt to bring up the blood pressure. The end result, however, is under-perfusion of liver, heart, brain, and kidneys.

Inflammatory mediators can be increased secondary to any type of tissue injury, inflammation of the body, or infectious process. Bacteria, for example, can release endotoxins that cause a compensatory release of inflammatory mediators (pro-inflammatory cytokines), including interleukin-1, tumor necrosis factor, and interleukin-6. Both phospholipid-derived mediators and cytokines act to change the microvascular permeability, the response of the microvasculature to vasoconstrictors (like norepinephrine), and cardiac function (by inhibiting the function of the myocytes). This results in an abnormal distribution of blood flow and tissue hypoxia.

There are problems with the coagulation cascade with regard to patients with distributive shock secondary to sepsis. Monocytes and endothelial cells become activated to cause an activation of the coagulation cascade (with involvement of cytokines). Antithrombin is impaired as is fibrinolysis. This results in disseminated intravascular coagulation or DIC, seen in up to 50 percent of patients with septicemia.

The decreased systemic vascular resistance (SVR) seen in anaphylactic shock is caused by a massive release of histamine from mast cells after being bound by IgE. The other contributing factor includes a release of prostaglandins. This causes vasodilation of the peripheral vasculature and hypotension. TSS can result from infection with Streptococcus pyogenes (group A Streptococcus) or Staphylococcus aureus.

Septic shock is most commonly caused by a chest infection but less frequent causes of sepsis are the abdomen and genitourinary tract. Most cases of shock are secondary to bacteria, with an equal frequency of Gram-positive and Gram-negative bacteria. Parasites, fungal organisms, and viruses are less likely to cause septic shock.

Shock secondary to adrenal insufficiency results from autoimmune destruction of the adrenal glands, surgical excision of the adrenal gland, hemorrhage damaging the adrenal glands, or infections that destroy these glands. High dose steroids can suppress the adrenal response when withdrawn and decreased pituitary gland function can cause adrenal insufficiency.

The death rate from septic shock is about 20-18 percent but can be improved by rapidly fixing the underlying problem. These patients need to be recognized as early as possible so as to treat the infection and improve tissue oxygenation. The mortality rate is much decreased if the diagnosis is made in the emergency room rather than later. Things that worsen the prognosis from septic shock include alcohol use, poor immune function, elevated lactate levels, Pseudomonas infections, older age, and the presence of positive blood cultures for bacteria.

The first goal of treatment is to treat the underlying cause and to use volume resuscitation to bring the blood pressure up. If this fails, vasopressors should be used. Both dopamine and norepinephrine are first-line agents for bringing up the blood pressure. Second-line vasopressors include phenylephrine, vasopressin, dobutamine, and epinephrine. Low dose dopamine can dilate the renal vasculature, resulting in better kidney perfusion in patients who don't need higher doses of the drug.

IV antibiotics are also extremely important. If no obvious source has been found, a first-line choice would be a third-generation cephalosporin (like ceftazidime, ceftriaxone, or ceftizoxime). An aminoglycoside should be added if the host is immunocompromised. IV drug users with sepsis should be treated empirically with nafcillin and an aminoglycoside. Pneumonias from the community should get ceftriaxone plus a macrolide, while hospital-acquired pneumonia sepsis cases should get a combination of piperacillin/tazobactam, levofloxacin, and an aminoglycoside.

Genitourinary sources of sepsis should be empirically treated with an aminoglycoside plus ampicillin. Abdominal septic cases should be treated with ampicillin or a third-generation cephalosporin, clindamycin or metronidazole, and an aminoglycoside. Cases of meningitis and sepsis should be empirically treated with ceftriaxone plus vancomycin. Skin infections leading to sepsis should be treated with nafcillin and toxic shock syndrome best responds to clindamycin IV.

If distributive shock is secondary to anaphylaxis, the best treatment is subcutaneous epinephrine repeated every 20 minutes. IV epinephrine can also be used if SQ epinephrine is unsuccessful. Added to this should be diphenhydramine, given intramuscularly or intravenously for angioedema or hives.

Key Takeaways

- The four main types of shock are hypovolemic, cardiogenic, distributive, and obstructive.

- Trauma is most likely to lead to hypovolemic shock.

- The mainstay of treatment for cardiogenic shock is cardiac reperfusion.

- The mainstay of treatment for septic shock is to treat the underlying infection while supporting the cardiovascular system.

Quiz

1. The patient has sustained a large anterior myocardial infarction. Statistically, what is the most prevalent cause of death in this type of patient?

   a. Congestive heart failure

   b. Ventricular wall rupture

   c. Cardiogenic shock

   d. Sudden cardiac arrhythmia

Answer: c. The most common cause of death secondary to a myocardial infarction is cardiogenic shock from pump failure.

2. You suspect that your patient has cardiogenic shock. What finding would you not expect to see with this type of diagnosis?

   a. Blood pressure less than 90 systolic

   b. Peripheral edema

   c. Cyanosis

   d. Muffled heart sounds

Answer: b. All of the following findings can be seen in patients who have cardiogenic shock with the exception of peripheral edema, which is not seen in the acute phases of this problem.

3. What would the most common clinical finding be to suggest poor perfusion of the kidneys?

   a. Hematuria

   b. Pyuria

   c. Bilateral flank pain

   d. Oliguria

Answer: d. The finding of oliguria strongly suggests poor perfusion of the kidneys so that little urine is made by these organs.

4. When the PAC is placed, it can determine the PCWP, which is also the same as what pressure measurement?

   a. Right atrial pressure

   b. Right ventricular pressure

   c. Left ventricular pressure

   d. Aortic pressure

Answer: c. The LV pressure is accurately measured by the determination of the PCWP in a PAC test.

5. What is not considered a typical electrolyte or acid-base problem in cardiogenic shock?

    a. Metabolic alkalosis

    b. Metabolic acidosis

    c. Hypokalemia

    d. Hypomagnesemia

Answer: a. All of the above are typical electrolyte findings in cardiogenic shock except for metabolic alkalosis.

6. For cardiogenic shock, what is the vasopressor of choice?

    a. Epinephrine

    b. Norepinephrine

    c. Dobutamine

    d. Dopamine

Answer: d. The treatment of choice is dopamine, which will increase blood pressure and improve renal blood flow.

7. Within what period of time from admission to the ED should a percutaneous coronary angioplasty be done to have the maximal effectiveness in cardiogenic shock?

    a. 30 minutes

    b. 90 minutes

    c. 240 minutes

    d. 360 minutes

Answer: b. The window of opportunity for a successful PCI procedure when the patient has a suspected coronary occlusion and cardiogenic shock is about 90 minutes after admission.

8. In giving inotropic and vasopressor agents to patients with cardiogenic shock, what mean arterial pressure or MAP should be the target level?

    a. Above 60 mm Hg

    b. Above 80 mm Hg

    c. Above 100 mm Hg

    d. Above 120 mm Hg

Answer: a. The MAP should be at least 60 mmHg and is the target level for adequate perfusion of the peripheral tissues.

9. What is the main advantage of using an IABP or intra-aortic balloon pump in patients at risk for cardiogenic shock?

   a. It increases the systolic blood pressure.

   b. It increase preload to the heart.

   c. It prevents aortic regurgitation.

   d. It reduces left ventricular afterload, improving heart function.

Answer: d. The main advantage of the IABP is to reduce left ventricular afterload, which improves cardiac function.

10. The patient has anaphylactic shock with urticaria. What is the treatment of choice for the urticaria?

   a. Norepinephrine

   b. Prednisone

   c. Dopamine

   d. Diphenhydramine

Answer; d. Diphenhydramine is the treatment of choice for urticaria in distributive shock secondary to anaphylaxis.

Chapter 3: Cardiac Resuscitation

Cardiac resuscitation is the general emergency response to a cardiac arrest situation, which, in turn, usually results from a severe myocardial infarction with a severe arrhythmia, although things like a pulmonary embolism, ventricular wall rupture, low potassium levels, heavy exercise, and major blood loss can cause a cardiac arrest. This chapter will discuss the phenomenon of the cardiac arrest as well as the emergency medical response to this type of catastrophic event.

Cardiac Arrest

A cardiac arrest involves a sudden drop in cardiac output, leading a loss of consciousness and a lack of breathing. Prior to the arrest, common symptoms include shortness of breath, chest pain, and nausea. It needs urgent emergency intervention within a few minutes or death of brain cells and irreversible death occurs.

As mentioned, coronary artery disease with an acute MI is the most common cause of death. The most common inherited cause of sudden cardiac death from an arrhythmia is long QT syndrome, followed by inherited atrial fibrillation, Brugada syndrome (which causes ventricular fibrillation), catecholaminergic polymorphic ventricular tachycardia (a calcium-channel disorder causing arrhythmias in exercise), and short QT syndrome.

The most common causes of structural hereditary cause of cardiac arrest are hypertrophic obstructive and nonobstructive cardiomyopathy (H[O]CM), arrhythmogenic right-ventricular cardiomyopathy/dysplasia (ARVC/D), dilated cardiomyopathy (DCM), and noncompaction cardiomyopathy.

For those arrest situations in which a rhythm strip can be obtained acutely, the most common arrhythmia found would be ventricular fibrillation, although, if time passes before the rhythm strip is obtained, the rhythm will degenerate into asystole. This problem occurs at a higher rate among people who smoke, live a sedentary lifestyle, or who are overweight.

The first-line treatment for a cardiac arrest is to assess the patient for shockable rhythm and defibrillate if a shockable rhythm is detected. This is shortly followed by cardiopulmonary resuscitation or CPR, which starts with cardiac compressions. CPR done by laypeople involves compression-only CPR, while CPR from a trained healthcare professional involves both compressions and artificial breathing/respirations. Patients who survive have the option of temperature management to improve CNS outcomes. Later, an implantable cardiac defibrillator may be used to prevent a recurrent event.

About 325,000 people in the US suffer an out-of-hospital cardiac arrest, while about 210,000 people have an arrest in the hospital. It is increasingly common with advanced age and happens more commonly in male. Those who are adequately treated have a survival chance of about 8 percent.

Symptoms of a Cardiac Arrest

Some people will have no symptoms preceding their arrest. Others will have chest pain, shortness of breath, dizziness, or vomiting. There may be a recent history of fainting spells or blackouts suggesting prior events. When the event does occur, the patient is nearly instantly unconscious and will have no palpable pulse. Breathing will stop and there will be a concomitant respiratory arrest.

Causes of Cardiac Arrest

The vast majority of cardiac arrest patients have coronary ischemia and suffer their arrest because of ventricular fibrillation (60-70 percent of cases). There is usually a high degree of blockage of at least one of the larger coronary arteries—as can be found on autopsy among those that die from the event. Another cause of sudden death is left ventricular hypertrophy secondary to long-term hypertension.

Low potassium and low magnesium levels account for a smaller proportion of cardiac arrest cases. Another thing that can be seen on autopsy besides a coronary occlusion is the finding of a recent myocardial infarction—seen in thirty percent of autopsies after SCD.

Among males aged 18-35, some type of structural heart abnormality is found in about half of all cases of SCD. A third of cases have no known etiology. Of known causes of structural heart disease, about 60 percent were found to have coronary arterial abnormalities, 20 percent had myocarditis, and 13 percent had hypertrophic cardiomyopathy. Having congestive heart failure was found to increase the risk of SCD by a factor of five.

About 35 percent of cases of sudden cardiac death are caused by a non-cardiac condition. The most common non-cardiac cause of a SCD is trauma. Secondary causes include some type of internal bleeding (GI tract, large vessel rupture, intracranial source), drowning, overdose, and pulmonary embolism. Rarely, poisoning or toxicities can cause a sudden cardiac death.

The diagnosis of cardiac arrest is primarily diagnosed by a lack of a carotid pulse. There are other findings that don't make the gold standard criterion for sudden cardiac death. These include unconsciousness, lack of movement, and a lack of breathing. Some patients can have a cardiac arrest but will still have agonal breathing.

A lack of breathing signifies a respiratory arrest but not a cardiac arrest and unconsciousness can occur in many other situations that do not qualify as a cardiac arrest.

A cardiac arrest can be determined as being "shockable" or "not shockable". This is completely determined by the ECG rhythm strip. A shockable rhythm can be treated with defibrillation, while a non-shockable rhythm will not be affected by defibrillation. The two main shockable rhythms include ventricular fibrillation and pulseless ventricular tachycardia. Some examples of non-shockable rhythms include pulseless electrical activity and asystole.

The Implantable Cardioverter Defibrillator in SCD

Patients who survive an out-of-hospital cardiac arrest can prevent further or repeated events. Placing an implantable cardioverter-defibrillator or ICD. This is implanted under the skin with electrodes attached to the heart. It does not have any pacemaker function; however, a pacemaker can be used with it.

Modern ICDs will detect a tachyarrhythmia and will deliver a synchronized cardioversion rather than just a defibrillation (which is non-synchronized). Patients who have had a cardiac arrest and are at risk for another cardiac arrest stand to benefit the most from an ICD placement.

Figure 7 shows a chest x-ray with a cardioverter defibrillator in place:

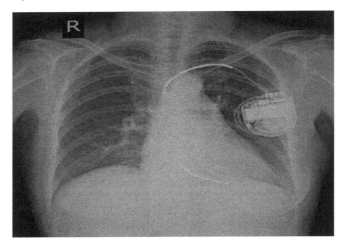

Figure 7

Management of a SCD Situation

There are several ways that a SCD situation is treated. All of these include some measure of resuscitation. In the field, resuscitation normally involves BLS or basic life support, which involves only some version of cardiopulmonary resuscitation or CPR. If a healthcare provider is adequately trained, the care of the patient can involve ACLS (Advanced Cardiac Life Support), which involves CPR, defibrillation, cardioversion, intubation, and medications. Children in an arrest situation are managed via PALS (Pediatric Advanced Life Support), while newborn resuscitation involves guidelines based on NRP or Neonatal Resuscitation Program.

Cardiopulmonary Resuscitation or CPR

CPR or cardiopulmonary resuscitation Is a crucial part of the cardiac arrest management. It should be begun a soon as the arrest is witnessed. Because chest compressions are the most effective part of CPR, it is considered the mainstay of the program. When correctly performed, CPR can improve the patient's survival rate but it is not correctly performed in more than 70 percent of cases. Resuscitation efforts should last about 20 minutes in asystole before determining that the patient isn't getting better, except in hypothermia or near-drowning situations.

Breathing can involve anything from a bag-valve mask (BVM), mouth-to-mouth resuscitation, or endotracheal intubation. The least likely method of providing ventilations is the surgical airway, which takes a great deal of expertise from a skilled provider. Endotracheal tube intubation, which is commonly-used, does not improve survival rates and may make it worse if done by inexperienced people.

The rate of compressions to ventilations is about 30 compressions to 2 ventilations. Bystander CPR currently involves compressions only as this has been found to lead to superior outcomes when compared to regular CPR. Mechanical compressions can be used but are not as effective as other types of compressions. If a pregnant woman fails to regain a pulse within four minutes of resuscitative efforts, an emergency Cesarean section should be performed.

Defibrillation is performed when a shockable rhythm is detected on the defibrillator. This would involve either pulseless ventricular tachycardia or ventricular fibrillation. When used in children, about 2-4 Joules per kilogram are recommended. Automated external defibrillation is used in the field as more and more of them are available in places like sports venues, airports, and shopping malls. They come with directions and are basically fool-proof.

Figure 8 shows defibrillation in action:

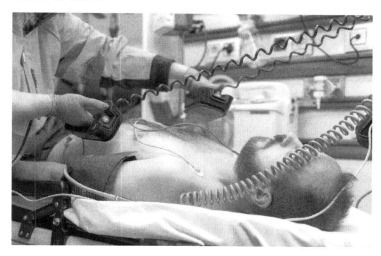

Figure 8

The use of ACLS means that medications will be given. The most common medication used in a cardiac arrest situation is epinephrine. Other choices include atropine, lidocaine, vasopressors, and amiodarone. Epinephrine has been found to maximize survival when given to patients in an arrest situation by intravenous or endotracheal means. Lidocaine and amiodarone are used in children. Sodium bicarbonate and calcium are usually not recommended in these cases.

Atropine should be used in bradycardic situations but it isn't used anymore in the treatment of asystole or pulseless electrical activity as it doesn't seem to be helpful. The same is true of giving amiodarone or lidocaine, which don't treat ventricular tachycardia or ventricular fibrillation, even if defibrillation is performed. Thrombolytics primarily are successful in situations where the pulmonary embolism is the cause of the SCD. Naloxone may be used if an opioid toxicity is felt to be the cause of the cardiac arrest.

One thing can be done after spontaneous circulation has been restored is to start a therapeutic hypothermia. This is especially true when consciousness has not been restored after the arrest. Patients are kept cool for one full day and have a target core temperature of 90-97 degrees Fahrenheit. This lowers the mortality rate by 30 percent and improves other outcomes. The earlier the cooling starts, the better the prognosis.

Some patients have a "do not resuscitate order" or DNR in their advanced health care directive, which indicate that they not be resuscitated if their heart stops. Patients may also indicate whether or not they want to be on a ventilator if they have a respiratory arrest or may ask only for comfort measures to be given in the situation of a terminal illness, allowing for a natural and comfortable death.

The things that provide for the best survival include early recognition of the pre-arrest signs and correcting underlying disease before the arrest occurs. Every minute after the arrest decreases the survival rate by 10 percent. Early CPR is also important as it improve blood flow and oxygen to the brain and other end organs. In shockable rhythms, ventricular fibrillation and pulseless ventricular tachycardia, early defibrillation will prolong survival rate. A soon as possible, advanced cardiac life support should be initiated along with definitive percutaneous coronary intervention or other type of revascularization procedure should they be warranted.

The use of the precordial thump is somewhat controversial. It should be considered in cases where the arrest was both monitored and witnessed, especially in pulseless VTach if a defibrillator is not immediately available. It shouldn't delay CPR or cardioversion.

Prognosis

The survival rate for an out-of-hospital cardiac arrest is about 7.6 percent, with survival rates among children approaching 16 percent. For in-hospital cardiac arrest, the survival rate is about 22 percent, with many having good CNS outcomes. Survival rates of a witnessed arrest is about 25 percent for out of hospital cardiac arrests. The survival rate decreases with age, at less than 20 percent in patients who have an in-hospital arrest after the age of 70 years. The survival rate of an out of hospital arrest to the time of discharge is about 6.8 percent. Of these 89 percent had normal brain function and 2 percent having a major neurological disability. Seventy percent of discharged persons are still alive after four years.

Complications of CPR

CPR is considered a last resort intervention is cases where the person will die without the procedure. Complications of CPR (even when done successfully) include rib fractures, fractures of the sternum, anterior mediastinal hemorrhaging, contusion of the heart, upper airway injuries, hemopericardium, pneumothorax, hemothorax, contusions of the young, and fat emboli. Of these, the most common complication from CPR is a rib fracture. The complication rate of this is between 13 percent and 97 percent. Sternal fractures have the second-highest complication rate.

In out of hospital cardiac arrests, the rate of attempted CPR in the US is between 14 and 45 percent (with an average of 32 percent. Some parts of the world have a CPR incidence of 1 percent per arrest. Only half of the time is this CPR performed correctly. Younger people are more likely to receive CPR before EMS services arrive at the scene. It is more common to have CPR begun outside the home when compared to an in-home SCD. Most responders in this situation are some type of healthcare provider. CPR should be started within six minutes of the arrest. Exceptions to this rule include near-drowning and hypothermia cases, which have survival rates that are good after several minutes without initiating CPR.

Key Takeaways

- The gold standard for a cardiac arrest is the absence of a carotid pulse.
- The survival rate from an out of hospital SCD is about 7 percent.
- The definitive treatment for a cardiac arrest is a revascularization procedure.
- The main cause of a cardiac arrest is an acute MI leading to ventricular fibrillation.

Quiz

1. In evaluating a person who has sustained an out-of-hospital cardiac arrest, what would you expect to be the most likely cause of this event?

   a. Traumatic blood loss

   b. Acute myocardial infarction

   c. Severe hypokalemia

   d. Acute heart failure

Answer: b. The most common cause of a cardiac arrest is a myocardial infarction leading to a nonperfusing cardiac arrhythmia.

2. What cardiac rhythm are you most likely find soon after a cardiac arrest?

   a. Asystole

   b. Supraventricular tachycardia

   c. Third-degree heart block

   d. Ventricular fibrillation

Answer: d. The most common cardiac arrhythmia found after an acute myocardial infarction and a cardiac arrest is ventricular fibrillation.

3. You have evaluated a young patient who has an inherited cause of a sudden cardiac death. What is the most common cause of an inherited arrhythmia causing a young person to have a cardiac arrest?

   a. Short QT syndrome

   b. Brugada syndrome

   c. Long QT syndrome

   d. Atrial fibrillation

Answer: c. The most common cause of an inherited arrhythmia leading to sudden cardiac death is long QT syndrome. The other choices are less common causes of an arrhythmia situation that is hereditary.

4. Which of the following cardiac rhythms is considered "shockable" in a cardiac arrest?

   a. Pulseless electrical activity

   b. Third degree heart block

   c. Asystole

   d. Pulseless ventricular tachycardia

Answer: d. Of the listed rhythms, the finding of pulseless ventricular tachycardia is considered a shockable rhythm.

5. What modern feature has been included in more recent ICDs that expand their usefulness?

   a. Detection of bradyarrhythmias

   b. Ability to detect PACs

   c. Ability for synchronized cardioversion

   d. Pacemaker capabilities

Answer: c. A more recent feature of ICDs is the ability to do synchronized cardioversion in cases of a tachyarrhythmia.

6. What is considered the most common cardiac/resuscitative protocol used in an out of hospital cardiac arrest?

   a. BLS

   b. ACLS

   c. PALS

   d. NRP

Answer: b. The most commonly used protocol for an out of hospital cardac arrest is basic life support or BLS.

7. Which type of ventilations are least likely to be used for patients needing CPR in the field?

   a. Mouth to mouth resuscitation

   b. BVM ventilations

   c. Endotracheal intubation

   d. Surgical airway ventilation

Answer: d. The least likely airway/ventilation technique is the surgical airway, which requires a well-trained individual to perform.

8. When using the automated external defibrillator and finding that it shocks the patient, what possible rhythm should be expected?

   a. Ventricular fibrillation

   b. Asystole

   c. Pulseless electrical activity

   d. Supraventricular tachycardia

Answer: a. Both pulseless ventricular tachycardia and ventricular tachycardia are considered shockable rhythms when detected by the AED device.

9. Which drug has been found to enhance the outcome of a cardiac arrest to the greatest degree?

    a. Atropine

    b. Amiodarone

    c. Bretylium

    d. Epinephrine

Answer: d. Epinephrine is the most common and the most effective drug in the treatment of cardiac arrest.

10. Which is considered the most common complication of CPR in adults?

    a. Rib fractures

    b. Sternal fractures

    c. Pneumothorax

    d. Cardiac contusion

Answer: a. Rib fracture happen in CPR in up to 97 percent of cases.

Chapter 4: Febrile Patient

One of the more common things an emergency medicine physician will have to deal with is the febrile patient. Most patients with fever will have some type of infection that needs to be discovered and managed. Less commonly, the cause of fever will be unrelated to an infection. This chapter focuses on the febrile patient, including the workup of fever, the diagnosis of fever, and the treatment of fever and febrile illnesses.

Causes of Fever

Fever actually starts in the hypothalamus of the brain, which is the thermostat or the organ that sets the body temperature of the body. When the thermostat causes an increase in temperature, the patient actually feels cold and will have chills. Chills will make a person shiver, which will further increase the body temperature. The body temperature is normally lower in the morning and higher in the evening. A normal body temperature is approximately 97°F to 99°F.

Causes of fever include a viral infection, a bacterial infection, heat exhaustion, autoimmune and inflammatory conditions, certain types of cancer, receiving immunizations, and certain medications. If the cause of the theater cannot be determined and the fever lasts for a prolonged period of time, the diagnosis is that of fever of unknown origin.

Fever in Children

Fever in children does not represent an illness but is instead the symptom of another physical problem. Most fevers in children are infectious in origin and most infections are viral. Fevers are part of the normal defense mechanism against infection. Other causes of a fever in a child include overdressing the child (particularly in babies), receiving immunizations, and teething. Not all fevers in children need to be treated with anything other than adequate hydration as it represents a normal defense mechanism that shouldn't be interfered with. Fevers that need treatment include a temperature that is greater than 102°F or a temperature greater than 104°F in an infant younger than three months of age. Fever in this age group may represent a serious illness and should be seen by the emergency room physician.

In an older child, signs of an unimportant fever include having a child that is still playing, is still eating and drinking appropriately, is alert and happy, has normal skin coloration, and otherwise appears well with a fever that easily goes down with an antipyretic drug.

The definition of a fever in a child includes the following:

1) an oral temperature greater than 100°F,

2) a rectal temperature of greater than 100.4°F, or

3) an axillary temperature of greater than 99°F. The actual elevation of the temperature isn't as important as the other physical findings; however, a very high fever should not be considered benign. Low body temperatures may be as significant in indicating an infection as a high body temperature.

Chills may also be a sign of a severe fever as this can raise the body temperature. Sweating tends to decrease the body temperature. A rapid respiratory rate is normal with a high fever but if the rapid respiratory rate persists after the fever is reduced, the parent should notify the child's physician or go to the emergency room.

The mainstay of treatment for a fever in children is Tylenol or acetaminophen. Another acceptable choice is ibuprofen. Both medications are given according to age or weight. Aspirin should never be given to a child because it can cause Reye syndrome, which can be fatal. No antipyretic drug should be given to infants under the age of two months without first checking with the emergency physician.

The febrile child may not eat well but they should be offered frequent liquids, including gelatin, ice pops, soup, and water so they can avoid the dehydration that comes frequently with the presence of a fever. Caffeinated beverages should be avoided as they cause diuresis and can increase boy fluid levels. The child with nausea, vomiting, and diarrhea should be offered an oral rehydration solution made for children. Sports drinks should be avoided as they make diarrhea worse. The sugars in fruit juices and fruits can make diarrhea worse.

Fever in the Older Adult

The older adult may not have the typical signs and symptoms seen in younger people. The normal basal body temperature decreases so smaller fevers may have more meaning in this population. They are also just as likely to be hypothermic with an infection, so low body temperatures need to be evaluated as well. Things that indicate the possibility of a fever being significant include a decline in functional status (such as new-onset confusion, falls, poor oral intake, belligerent behaviors, incontinence, and decreased mobility).

The definition of a fever in an older adult is one single oral temperature reading of greater than 100 degrees Fahrenheit, two oral temperature readings of greater than 99 degrees Fahrenheit, or two rectal temperatures of greater than 99.5 degrees Fahrenheit. In addition, fever can be defined as an increase in any type of temperature reading that is more than two degrees Fahrenheit over the baseline body temperature.

Fever Evaluation

The first evaluation necessary in the febrile older patient is to look for a source of an infection. This involves looking for ways that an infection can occur. Things like respiratory rate, hydration status, and mental status can tell if the cause of the fever is serious or not. Sources of a fever (in no particular order) include the oropharynx, skin (in all places of the body), conjunctiva, heart, lungs, abdomen, and any indwelling devices that may be present.

In part, the advanced directives given by the resident should direct the workup given to identify the source of the fever. Some nursing home residents (or the elderly person living in the nursing home) have specific directives against doing laboratory workups for febrile illnesses, with the expectation that any infection be treated only symptomatically without the goal being treatment or a cure for the underlying condition.

The first test that should be done is a CBC with differential (particularly focused on a manual differential that can assess the peripheral smear for band forms or immature WBCs). This should be done within 12-24 hours of the onset of a fever or sooner if the patient is seriously ill with symptoms related to a severe infection or complications of a fever. The presence of a WBC count greater than 14,000 or the presence of a left shift (with a band percentage of 6 percent or more) indicates the possibility of a bacterial infection, even if there is no fever. Without a fever, leukocytosis, or left shift, the presence of a bacterial infection is unlikely and further evaluation is unwarranted.

The second most-common test performed is a urinalysis or urine culture, which should be performed mainly on those elderly persons with an indwelling catheter or those who have symptoms of a urinary tract infection. A UA may be adequate in a person living in the community but there are a lot of resistant organisms in a nursing home setting so a urine culture may be an important part of the evaluation.

Indwelling catheters are particularly likely sources for urinary tract infections. Evidence of urosepsis with delirium, hypotension, shaking chills, or fever point to the possibility of urine being the source of the infection so a urine specimen should be collected along with an evaluation of the blood with a blood culture. An accurately collected urine specimen involves a clean-catch, midstream collection. If a woman requires a catheter specimen, it should be in-and-out and should be done using a technique that as sterile as possible. Indwelling catheters should be changed after recognition of a urinary source of infection.

At a minimum, a UTI evaluation should involve a urine dipstick that looks for nitrites and leukocyte esterase. If the dipstick shows positivity of either of these, a microscopic urinalysis should be done. If this shows pyuria or bacteriuria, a urine culture should be performed. In addition, if urosepsis is suspected, both blood and urine cultures with sensitivity testing should be done as well as a Gram stain of an uncentrifuged sample of urine.

Blood Culture Evaluations

Blood cultures of the febrile older patient are not generally recommended as they provide a very low yield and do not often influence the course of therapy. If bacteremia is highly suspected, however, and if there is an easy access to laboratory resources for blood culture assessment, it may be something worthwhile doing, especially if a source of infection and other areas of possible culturing are unavailable.

Figure 9 shows an aerobic blood culture vessel:

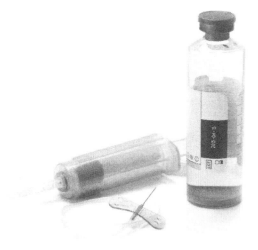

Figure 9

Evaluation of the Febrile Patient with Possible Pneumonia

If the adult/elderly patient has a clinically-suspected case of pneumonia, the following tests ae worthwhile doing: 1) a pulse oximetry reading if the patient has an elevated respiratory rate in order to see if the patient is hypoxic. The presence of hypoxia may tip the scales toward the possibility of oxygen therapy and a transfer to a hospital setting, particularly if there are no oxygen sources in the home or nursing facility.

A chest x-ray is the second test that should be performed if hypoxia is present in order to look for the presence of an infiltrate compatible with acute pneumonia. The other goal of the chest x-ray is to exclude things like a mass in the lungs, concomitant heart failure, pleural effusions, or multi-lobular pneumonia.

If the infection is suspected to be viral, swabs should be taken from the throat and nasopharynx from both the suspected patient and any other acutely ill patients living with the target patient so that a rapid diagnostic test should be performed for influenza A. This is treatable with antiviral medications so it is important to isolate an influenza A outbreak and treat cases as early as possible. Outbreaks of other viruses can be tested for and treated if possible.

Evaluation of Skin and Soft Tissue Infections

These can be evaluated and treated on clinical grounds with no need for a tissue culture or a surface swab culture as most cases come from streptococcus or staphylococcus species. The biggest exception is a conjunctival infection, which should be swabbed and cultured. Deep tissue biopsies or needle aspiration can be done in cases where a fluctuant abscess is present, unusual pathogens are expected, or if initial antimicrobial therapy fails.

If there is an expected pressure ulcer infection that doesn't seem to heal or has persistent purulent drainage, deep tissue specimens of the tissue should be obtained. Bone tissue should be looked at as sources of deep infection if the ulcer is overlying bone. The best way to assess the patient for osteomyelitis is to obtain an MRI evaluation, which is the most sensitive way to detect infection in the bony tissue. If this is positive, a bone biopsy should be done to look for an organism or organisms (and to get a culture).

If the skin infection is suspected to be fungal in origin, a skin scraping test can be done with a KOH smear to check for dermatophytes or yeast. If empiric treatment fails in suspected candidiasis cases, a culture should be done to look for the possibility of drug-resistant cases that haven't responded to the most likely antimicrobial agents.

If the patient clinically is suspected to have a herpes zoster infection or herpes simplex infection, a skin scraping looking for giant cells (which is called a Tzanck preparation) and a viral culture can be obtained. If this is not possible, a viral antigen test (an immunofluorescent test) or a polymerase chain reaction (PCR) test can be done on the blood.

In a setting where a generalized rash that is pruritic is found in an elderly patient who might be exposed to scabies, a light microscopy evaluation of a skin scraping with mineral oil should be done, looking for the mites themselves, the eggs, or the feces from the organism. If this is positive for any of these things, the patient can be treated with antimicrobial lotion against scabies.

The Febrile Patient with GI Disease

Without any obvious gastrointestinal infection stemming from an outbreak in the community, the stable gastroenteritis patient can be monitored for up to a week with only ongoing evaluation of their fluid status. No cultures or bloodwork need to be performed unless the patient doesn't recover within a week or is extremely ill. In such a situation, protozoal species (including Giardia) should be looked for in a stool O and P evaluation.

If there is a severely high fever, abdominal pain, and either WBCs or blood in the stool, the first test that should be performed should be an evaluation for Clostridium difficile, particularly if antibiotics have been used within the prior month. Stool should be evaluated, looking for the C. difficile toxin. This may have to be repeated more than once if the infection is suspected but the initial test is negative.

In cases where the C. difficile toxin assay is negative and there is no recent history of antibiotic use, patients with bloody diarrhea, abdominal cramps, and fever should have a stool culture. The most common organisms suspected in such cases include Salmonella, Campylobacter, Shigella, and E. coli (type O157:H7). These can be cultured in the stool and can be effectively treated.

Less commonly, the source of the abdominal infection will not involve the small or large bowel but will be an intrabdominal abscess. These infections are not common but will cause abdominal pain, high fever, and possible secondary septicemia. There is a great deal of morbidity and mortality associated with these types of infections and things like a CT scan of the abdomen, ultrasound of the abdomen, or an MRI of the abdomen are the best way of identifying these infections so they can be drained and treated with antibiotics.

When should a Fever be further Evaluated?

Some fevers are completely benign, while others are dangerous and should be evaluated and treated. Any fever greater than 104 degrees Fahrenheit in either children or adults needs further evaluation. A child under the age of three months with a fever of greater than 100.4 degrees Fahrenheit rectally should be evaluated. All patients with AIDS, cancer, heart disease, diabetes, or immunosuppression should be evaluated further to find an underlying cause for their fever.

Any child with a fever that has other signs and symptoms suggestive of severity, such as sore throat, stiff neck, unusual rash, ear pain, headache or fussiness should be seen. A child under two years of age with fever lasting more than one day should be seen as should any child over the age of two with fever lasting more than three days.

A febrile patient should be monitored for evidence of severe disease, such as stiff neck, confusion, and somnolence (indicative of meningitis), flank pain, shaking chills, and dysuria (indicative of pyelonephritis), shortness of breath or cough (indicative of pneumonia), or things like abdominal pain, tenderness to the abdomen, nausea, vomiting, and diarrhea (seen in abdominal infections). Certain skin rashes can be a sign of a number of infectious diseases (like Rocky Mountain spotted fever, rheumatic fever, chicken pox, or scarlet fever).

The finding of fever blisters is not serious but are small vesicles and ulcerations that occur on the mouth, lips, and tongue of patients who first get a herpes simplex virus (usually the first-time infection). These can be very severe, interfering with eating and drinking.

Pregnant women with a fever of greater than 101 degrees Fahrenheit should be seen by the doctor, especially when it is associated with joint pain and a rash. Serious febrile infections that can adversely affect the baby include rubella, cytomegalovirus, and Zika virus infections. Simple colds or flus in pregnancy can be treated mainly by managing the fever.

A small percentage of children and toddlers under the ages of three years will have a febrile seizure at least once in their lives. It has been estimated that one in every 25 children will experience at least one febrile seizure during their childhood, usually on the first day of their fever. While these are dramatic complications of fevers, they do not lead to long-term complications and do not need to be treated with anti-epileptic drugs. Later development of epilepsy occurs more frequently in children who have had febrile seizures; however, the risk that a child will develop epilepsy after a single febrile seizure is only slightly higher than that of a child who has never had a febrile seizure.

Key Takeaways

- Fever in children is generally benign but should be taken seriously among children under three months of age.

- There are specific ways of interpreting the temperature in the febrile child and adult.

- Older adults also have the potential to have fevers for infectious and non-infectious reasons.

- There are specific workups for the febrile adult that depend on the other findings seen in these patients.

- Febrile seizures are common in toddlers and don't always predict later onset of epilepsy.

Quiz

1. Fevers can be of many different origins. What is least likely to be a cause of fever in an adult patient?

    a. Malignancy

    b. Rheumatological disease

    c. Bacterial infection

    d. Blood loss

Answer: d. All of the above can be causes of a fever except for blood loss, which does not result in a fever.

2. You are evaluating the fever in a 2-year-old child. What sign would least likely give you the impression that this is a benign fever?

    a. Fever of 104.4 degrees Fahrenheit axillary

    b. Reduction fever to normal after receiving an antipyretic drug

c. Evidence of mild dehydration

d. The absence of nausea and vomiting

Answer: a. A fever that is as high as 104.4 degrees Fahrenheit is least associated with a benign fever.

3. What medication is the mainstay of treatment for fever in a child?

a. Ibuprofen

b. Naproxen

c. Acetaminophen

d. Aspirin

Answer: c. Acetaminophen is the treatment of choice in the febrile child with a benign or non-benign fever.

4. In evaluating a patient whom you suspect has urosepsis, what is the best way to determine if this is the case?

a. Blood culture for Gram-negative organisms

b. Urine culture

c. CBC with differential

d. Urine dipstick

Answer: d. The test of choice is a urine dipstick, which will quickly show a positive leukocyte esterase or positive nitrite test if the urine is the source of the infection. If both of these are negative, further testing for a urinary source of infection does not need to happen.

5. In caring for the patient suspected of having pneumonia, what is the definitive test in determining the course of action taken to treat this problem?

a. Pulse oximetry reading on room air

b. Chest x-ray

c. Sputum cytology

d. CBC with differential

Answer: a. The pulse oximetry reading will determine whether or not the patient is hypoxic and will direct whether the patient can be treated at home or needs a hospital admission for oxygen therapy and parenteral antibiotics.

6. Which soft tissue infections should be immediately cultured before treating with antibiotics?

a. Lower extremity infections

b. Infections in diabetic patients

c. Conjunctival infections

d. Lymph node infections

Answer: c. When it comes to soft tissue infections, the main infections that should be cultured before treating include conjunctival infections, which should be swabbed.

7. What is the preferred test to do on a patient suspected of having a febrile illness secondary to a herpes simplex infection of the skin?

   a. Tzanck smear

   b. Polymerase chain reaction

   c. Viral antigen load of the blood

   d. Viral blood culture

Answer: a. A Tzanck smear of the skin will show giant cells in cases of a herpes simplex infection, which will lead to a fast diagnosis of a viral herpes infection.

8. You are caring for a patient who has had gastroenteritis with watery diarrhea for a week. This is an adult patient who has a low-grade fever and does not have any affected contacts in their life. What should you order to evaluate this febrile patient?

   a. CBC with differential

   b. Stool sample for ova and parasites

   c. Blood culture

   d. Stool culture

Answer: b. The clinical picture is inconsistent with a bacterial infection of the GI tract so the test of choice would be to evaluate the patient for a protozoal infection, such as Giardia. The diagnostic test of choice would be a stool sample for ova and parasites.

9. You are managing the care of an adult who was on a 3-week course of antibiotics for chronic sinusitis and who developed bloody diarrhea, crampy abdominal pain, and fever. What test might best help diagnose the cause of this abdominal infection?

   a. Stool culture

   b. Blood culture

   c. Stool sample for ova and parasites

   d. Stool sample for C. difficile toxin

Answer: d. The clinical course is suspicious for C. difficile. A culture will not be helpful and an ova and parasite examination will likely be negative. At least one stool sample for Clostridium difficile toxin should be assayed before antibiotic therapy is started against the organism.

10. Which of the following infectious, febrile illnesses in pregnancy will least likely lead to birth defects?

a. Zika fever

b. Influenza A

c. Rubella

d. Cytomegalovirus

Answer: b. Influenza A is least likely to cause birth defects in a pregnant mother who contracts the disease. The others carry the potential of birth defects when the pregnant woman develops the infection.

Chapter 5: Chest Pain

Chest pain in the adult emergency department patient can be serious or benign but always need to be worked up by the emergency room physician in order to identify which types of chest pain need further intervention and which can simply be monitored. This chapter discusses the phenomenon of chest pain and the possible things that can cause this important symptom.

Causes of Chest Pain

Research has been performed on the major causes of chest pain in the emergency room population. According to the latest studies, about 36 percent of chest pain is purely musculoskeletal in origin (related to chest wall pain), gastrointestinal in 19 percent of cased, nonspecific in 16 percent of cases, stable angina in 10 percent of cases, psychogenic in origin 7 percent of the time, respiratory in origin 5 percent of the time, and related to unstable ischemic heart problems 1.5 percent of the time. Non-ischemic heart conditions account for 4 percent of cases of chest pain.

The least serious causes of chest pain are musculoskeletal and include Tietze syndrome, costochondritis, and costosternal syndrome. Age and gender play no roles in deciding if the patient has a chest wall cause for their chest pain. The main findings are an absence of a cough or other respiratory symptoms, pain that is sharp or stinging, pain that is reproducible on touching the chest, and secondary muscle tension.

On the other side of the spectrum are patients who might have an acute MI as a cause of their chest pain. There is a simple scoring system that leads to the possibility that the pain is cardiac in origin. These give one point to each of the following risk factors: Age older than 55 years in males and 65 years in females, known CAD or past stroke, non-reproducible pain, pain increasing with exercise, and the assumption by the patient that the pain is cardiogenic in origin. Patients with all of these features had an 11-fold incidence in having their chest pain caused by myocardial ischemia.

Electrocardiographic findings (ECG findings) can also lead to a diagnosis of an acute MI. The most common predictors of an acute MI as a cause of chest pain include ST segment elevation, new onset left bundle branch block, and hyperacute T waves. Other findings are less suggestive of an MI when an ECG is obtained on the chest pain patient.

If nonspecific ECG changes are found, other things can suggest an acute MI as a cause of the chest pain. These include male gender, older age (more than 60 years), pressure-like chest pain, and pain radiation to the back, jaw, neck, or arm). A patient with none of these clinical findings has less than a 1 percent chance of having an acute myocardial infarction.

Basic Workup of Chest Pain

The first step in working up chest pain is to determine the risk factors for coronary artery disease. Low risk patients, scoring 0 or 1 on the above criteria measurements should first be evaluated for noncardiac chest pain unless there are physical findings suggestive of heart disease. Moderate risk patients should have an ECG and a determination of whether or not ischemic changes are found. If there are ischemic changes, a serum troponin level should be drawn to evaluate the possibility of cardiac necrosis. If there are nonspecific changes, non-ischemic heart problems should be looked for. High risk patients should have an ECG performed and should be treated presumptively for having an MI with aspirin and cardiology referral.

Chest Wall Pain

Chest wall pain or musculoskeletal chest pain is the most common cause of chest pain in adults who present to the emergency department. There are many causes of musculoskeletal chest wall pain, most of which are relatively benign. In addition, most of these causes are completely self-limited and require no specific treatment except for pain relief. These are the more common causes of musculoskeletal chest wall pain:

- **Chest trauma**—a sprain or strain secondary to a fall can cause chest pain. In addition, there can be bruising of the ribs or fractured ribs caused by a car accident or more serious injury. In some cases, just lifting something heavy can strain the chest wall.

- **Costochondritis**—this is an inflammation of the anterior chest wall that is also referred to as costosternal syndrome or anterior chest wall syndrome. The location of the pain is the costochondral junction, which is the place where the ribs connect to the sternum in the anterior part of the chest. The pain is reproducible to palpation and can be on either side of the chest. Despite the name, there is no actual inflammation going on in the chest wall. Subtle dislocation of the ribs may be the cause of this problem.

- **Lower rib pain syndrome**—this is also referred to as "slipping rib syndrome". The pain is in the lower chest wall or abdomen. It occurs secondary to a loosening of the lower ribs from the cartilage that connects them to the sternum. This causes rib movement and pain that is reproducible by palpating the rib connection. It can be treated conservatively or surgically.

- **Precordial catch pain**—this is a sudden sharp chest pain seen in young people at rest. The pain is worse with breathing and, after a few minutes, goes away spontaneously. No one knows what causes this problem and it isn't known if it is significant.

- **Fibromyalgia**—this is a more common condition of chest pain in middle-aged women. The pain isn't located just in the chest but is found all over the body. It is associated with other systemic findings, like GI symptoms, sleep disorder, and overall fatigue. The exact cause of the problem is not felt to be an actual inflammation but an abnormal response to pain receptors in the chest wall.

- **Rheumatoid conditions**—these types of pain are associated with spinal or rib joint inflammation. The rheumatoid problems most linked to this type of pain are psoriatic arthritis, ankylosing spondylitis, and rheumatoid arthritis. Usually, other joints are affected besides the rib-sternal joints.

- **Stress fractures**—this is generally a repetitive stress injury seen in athletes who engage in repetitive stress involving the upper arms, such as seen in baseball pitchers and rowers. It tends to be worse in people who have vitamin D deficiency states or osteoporosis.

- **Cancer**—certain types of cancer can lead to chest wall pain, primarily breast cancer or lung cancer. It is rare to have bone cancer primarily affecting the ribs but metastatic bone cancer can have metastases to the bones of the chest wall.

- **Sickle cell crisis**—this is found in people with sickle cell disease who have small infarctions of the ribs from sickling of the blood cells. This causes chest pain that is relatively self-limiting.

The main treatment for musculoskeletal chest is to treat the pain and underlying condition. NSAIDs are more likely to lead to help this type of pain over any other type of pain-reliever, such as acetaminophen or narcotic pain medications.

Acute Coronary Syndrome

This is perhaps the most severe cause of chest pain. The diagnosis is made quickly by an ECG showing a STEMI (ST-segment elevation acute myocardial infarction) but the ECG shows this in only a small percentage of chest pain patients. Things that can present with similar symptoms to acute coronary syndrome (ACS) include GERD, pleural irritation, pericarditis, pulmonary embolism, hyperventilation, cholecystitis, and chest wall pain.

The biggest challenge is to identify these patients correctly so as to treat them as soon as possible while avoiding unnecessary testing and intervention in patients who do not have ACS. There are high medical costs in treating ACS so it should be avoided in patients who don't have the disease.

Another testing modality available to identify the patient with ACS is blood testing for myocardial markers. The absence of these markers being positive doesn't exclude ACS in some cases. The serum troponin level is the most often used test to see if ACS is present; however, other serum markers, such as CPK-MB, LDH, and AST can be elevated.

Because the diagnosis of ACS can be difficult, there are several risk scores that have been identified to find patients that have the greatest risk for ACS (and a poor outcome) and who would most benefit from aggressive interventions.

One scoring system is the PURSUIT score that was developed to identify those patients with unstable angina. It looked at several parameters, giving points for things like age, history of recent angina, gender, ST segment depression on ECG, and evidence of heart failure. Things like hypotension and tachycardia were not included in the scoring table as they weren't predictors of death or MI at thirty days after the emergency visit. Low risk patients can be discharged with observation only, while high risk patients are directed toward aggressive therapies.

The TIMI risk score is another way of identifying patients with likely ACS. The risk score gave point to those having an age greater than 65 years, recent angina use, recent known angina, at least three risk factors for CAD, known CAD by angiography, elevated cardiac markers on presentation, and deviation in the ST segment (high or low by more than 0.5 mm). A high score predicts all-cause mortality, the presence of ACS, or recurrent ischemia in the next 14 days requiring a revascularization procedure.

The GRACE scoring system looked at risk factors for in-hospital death and post-discharge death at six months after onset of chest pain. The risk factors looked at were the Killip class for CHF, elevated systolic BP, advanced age, creatinine level in the blood, cardiac arrest at the time of admission, ST-segment deviations, and increased cardiac enzyme levels. High risk patients had the highest risk of in-hospital death and death within six months of onset of chest pain. In fact, high risk patients had a greater than 50 percent risk of in-hospital death.

The FRISC scoring system predicted death and myocardial infarction in patients with evidence of unstable angina at the time of presentation. The risk score was confined to age greater than 70 years, male gender, diabetes, previous myocardial infarction, ST segment depression, elevated troponin I level, and elevated interleukin-6 or CRP level. The maximum total score is 7 points. High risk patients had a higher risk of death from myocardial infarction. Patients with a FRISC score of at least three points are recommended to have early intervention for probable CAD and ACS.

The HEART scoring system is designed to evaluate patients presenting for emergency evaluation of chest pain. This gives points to patients with a past history of angina, advanced age, risk factors for ACS, ECG findings, and troponin level. High risk patients had a higher risk of their chest pain being secondary to MI and to need percutaneous coronary intervention at the time of admission. Patients scoring 7-10 on a 10-point scale had a 65 percent chance of an MI, while patients scoring 0-3 had a 0.9 percent chance of an MI.

Treatment of ACS

Once the ACS patient is identified, he or she needs to be treated. The focus is on stabilizing their vital signs, relieving pain, and unblocking the affected arteries to reduce the degree of myocardial damage. Morphine or fentanyl can be given for pain control, oxygen is provided, patients are given nitroglycerin, aspirin is given, and clopidogrel is given as soon as the diagnosis is made. Nitrates are not indicated in complete vessel occlusion.

Patients with NSTEMI ACS need urgent treatment with aspirin, heparin (low molecular weight heparin or regular heparin), clopidogrel, IV platelet glycoprotein IIb/IIIa complex inhibitors and beta blockers. A second-line treatment is revascularization when they are stabilized with the above medications. Low risk patients should have a biomarker evaluation looking for evidence of myocardial muscl infarction. Even low risk patients seem to benefit from clopidogrel treatment.

Nitrates cannot be given for right ventricular infarctions, hypotensive patients, severe aortic stenosis, large pericardial effusion, or those who recently took sildenafil or another phosphodiesterase-5 inhibitor. They can be given in all other situations to dilate the vasculature and improve coronary blood flow.

An intra-aortic balloon pump is necessary in cases where the patient is hypotensive or has intractable chest pain. There is a 40 percent reduction in the risk of death among these types of patients who have the IABP placed. The use of this device supports the patient's heart function until they resolve their infarction complications.

Patients with cardiogenic shock have the highest mortality rate after an MI and need things like dobutamine and dopamine, as well as percutaneous intervention or CABG to improve their coronary artery ischemia. Stent thrombosis can always occur after PCI and poses a risk for another myocardial infarction which might require treatment with another PCI or CABG.

Nitrates have been found to decrease ischemic pain but don't improve the mortality rate. They do improve collateral blood flow, improve coronary vasodilation, decrease afterload, and decrease preload. They should be avoided in hypotensive patients as they can make hypotension worse.

Beta blockers are first-line treatments for all patients with myocardial infarction unless they have certain contraindications, such as systolic BP less than 90 mm Hg, severe bradycardia, cardiogenic shock, second- or third-degree heart block, or a lung condition that might be made worse with beta-agonist therapy. Patients with uncompensated CHF or peripheral vascular disease shouldn't have beta blocker therapy either.

Beta blockers decrease myocardial oxygen demand and decrease the incidence of adverse heart events and overall mortality. They prevent papillary muscle ruptures, ruptures of the left ventricle, and ruptures of the ventricular septum. The most commonly used beta-blocker intervention is IV metoprolol, given every five minutes until 15 mg total is given. As mentioned, they can't be used in cardiogenic shock or in patients with evidence of heart failure at the time of presentation.

Antiplatelet Drugs

Aspirin is an antiplatelet drug indicated for ACS patients as a first-line agent. It blocks the cyclooxygenase pathway of thromboxane A2 production in platelets so that the platelets won't aggregate. It is given as soon as ACS is suspected and continued for the duration of the patient's life, reducing overall morbidity and mortality from cardiovascular disease.

Clopidogrel goes by the generic name thienopyridine. It blocks the adenosine 5'-diphosphate (ADP)-dependent activation of the glycoprotein IIb/IIIa complex, which is an important step in platelet aggregation. As an antiplatelet drug, it is a first-line treatment for suspected ACS patients. It is especially useful when given along with aspirin, reducing the rate of an infarction by 20 percent. It is often withheld until after the PCA (percutaneous angiography) because it can't be used for five days prior to a CABG procedure. Clopidogrel can be a good alternative to aspirin therapy in patients who are allergic to aspirin or who can't for some other reason take aspirin therapy. The major complication of clopidogrel therapy is gastrointestinal bleeding. For this reason, it should be used with caution in patients who have a past GI bleeding history, an H. pylori infection, NSAID therapy, or steroid therapy. Proton pump inhibitor therapy has been found to reduce the risk of GI bleeding in patients on clopidogrel.

Prasugrel is another thienopyridine ADP receptor blocker that inhibits the aggregation of platelets. It reduces the incidence of both first and recurrent MIs. It is given as a first-line therapy in suspected ACS patients and reduces complications of PCI, such as stent thrombosis. Like clopidogrel, it should be postponed until after the angiogram in case the patient is only a candidate for the CABG procedure. There are more bleeding complications with prasugrel but the overall mortality rate is the same as with clopidogrel.

A newer drug called vorapaxar is indicated in ACS patients as it reduces the risk of stroke, another MI, and the need for revascularization in patients with chest pain from ACS (or those with PAD). It is an anti-platelet drug that blocks platelet aggregation by acting as a proteas-activated receptor 1 (PAR-1) blocker. It is used along with aspirin and clopidogrel in patients with ACS in the emergency room. It causes severe bleeding complications in 3.4 percent of patients who received the drug.

Another antiplatelet drug is ticagrelor, which is a reversible antiplatelet drug that seems to provide better ADP-receptor inhibition when compared to clopidogrel. Like clopidogrel, it reduces the rate of all-cause mortality in patients receiving the drug when given in the emergency department after evaluating the high-risk patient with probable ACS. As with all drugs of this type, there is a higher than normal risk of bleeding complications but they aren't generally fatal. It also seems to prevent stent thrombosis in those patients who have a stent placed.

Anticoagulation Therapy

There are several anticoagulation drugs that can be given to probable acute MI patients who have chest pain. One drug is unfractionated heparin, which has been found to reduce the risk of death by 33 percent, especially when given along with aspirin as an antiplatelet drug. It carries the risk of PCI bleeding around the time of the procedure and causes bleeding at the vascular access site so it should be used with bleeding complications in mind.

Factor Xa inhibitors seem to decrease mortality in patients with ACS. The drug most commonly used is rivaroxaban, which decreases the risk of death and bleeding complications after a diagnosis of ACS. Low-dose therapy has fewer complications with the same efficacy as high-dose therapy.

Another way of managing the ACS patient is to give thrombolytic therapy with tissue plasminogen activator. The sooner it is given, the less the risk of major cardiac muscle ischemia and necrosis. Its primary use is in the treatment of ACS when PCI procedures can't be performed or if there will be a delay in doing a PCI procedure. If the prehospital ECG shows a STEMI and PCI cannot be performed, this is the treatment of choice.

Coronary Interventions in ACS

All patients who have unstable angina or NSTEMI infarcts should have a revascularization procedure that starts with an angiogram with intent to do a PCI if indicated. This is the definitive treatment for all patients who have the availability of revascularization procedure resources. Early invasive therapy should also be considered in patients with a probable large infarct, hypotension, cardiogenic shock, refractory and ongoing chest pain despite medical therapy, and right ventricular infarction.

Current recommendations are that moderate-risk patients or high-risk patients with ACS have a combination of unfractionated or low-molecular-weight heparin therapy, aspirin, clopidogrel, and some type of PCI procedure. Some studies also indicate that glycoprotein IIb/IIIa inhibitors be used at the time of angiography but the risk of bleeding at the time of angiography is high and there is no evidence that they improve outcome.

Key Takeaways

- Chest pain is most likely to be musculoskeletal although there are several other types of problems that can present with chest pain, some of which are severe.

- Chest wall pain is most likely to be benign and self-limited and is usually a reproducible pain.

- Patients with ACS represent the far end of the morbidity spectrum and need early/aggressive treatment in order to manage their ischemia and chest pain.

Quiz

1. In evaluating the chest pain patient in the emergency room, it should be noted that the most common cause of chest pain in all patients is what?

   a. Musculoskeletal

   b. Gastrointestinal sources

   c. Stable angina

d. Acute myocardial infarction

Answer: a. Up to a third or more of all cases of chest pain are musculoskeletal in nature, representing mainly chest wall pain.

2. Which of the following chest pain scenarios is the most serious?

   a. Costochondritis

   b. Costosternal syndrome

   c. Tietze syndrome

   d. Pleural effusion

Answer: d. The first three choices are purely chest wall-related pain, which are extremely benign cases of chest pain. A pleural effusion is considered a more severe cause of chest pain.

3. In identifying a high-risk patient for chest pain secondary to myocardial ischemia, the biggest risk factors include all of the following but what?

   a. Personal history of acute MI or stroke

   b. Reproducible pain on palpation

   c. Belief by the patient that the pain is cardiac in origin

   d. Male age greater than 55 years and female age greater than 65 years

Answer: b. All of the above are predictors of cardiac chest pain except for having reproducible pain, which is not a risk factor for coronary-related pain.

4. You find that a patient has a cancerous lesion of the chest wall causing chest pain. Prior to doing a biopsy, what would the least likely place be for a primary cancer?

   a. Bone

   b. Brain

   c. Lung

   d. Breast

Answer: b. The least likely place for a metastatic lesion to the chest wall is brain cancer. The other choices are most likely to lead to metastatic lesions to the chest wall.

5. What is the most common ECG finding that is definitely confirmatory of ACS?

   a. ST segment depression

   b. PR interval shortening

   c. Inversion of the T wave

   d. ST segment elevation

Answer: d. ST segment elevation is a definite finding in STEMI, making it the most obvious way to diagnose acute coronary syndrome.

6. What is the most often-used cardiac marker used in the diagnosis of ACS?

    a. AST

    b. CPK-MB

    c. Troponin I

    d. LDH

Answer: c. The troponin I test is the main way to diagnose ACS in patients who have chest pain as it is positive shortly after myocardial tissue infarction.

7. Which patients have the worst prognosis after a myocardial infarction?

    a. Patients with three-vessel disease

    b. Patients who require a CABG versus a PCI procedure

    c. Patients with cardiogenic shock

    d. Patients aged 65 years or older

Answer: c. Patients with the worst prognosis have cardiogenic shock after a myocardial infarction, with an up to 90 percent mortality rate.

8. What cannot be said to be true of nitrate therapy in the treatment of chest pain patients with ACS?

    a. It causes arterial vasodilation.

    b. It reduces hypertension.

    c. It reduces ischemic pain.

    d. It improves mortality rates after an MI.

Answer: d. It does all of the above things in ACS but had not been found to improve the mortality rate.

9. You are anticipating giving a beta-blocker to a patient who has chest pain secondary to ACS. Which patient would least likely be a candidate for beta-blocker therapy?

    a. A patient with a BP of 140 systolic

    b. A patient with a second-degree heart block

    c. A patient with an inferior MI

    d. A patient with a heart rate of 80 bpm.

Answer: b. All of the above patients are candidates for beta-blocker therapy except for the patient with a second-degree heart block.

10. Patients with ACS should have early intensive treatment of their chest pain and ischemia. Which intervention is least likely to be helpful in these patients?

    a. Aspirin

    b. Clopidogrel

    c. Low molecular weight heparin

    d. Glycoprotein IIb/IIIa inhibitors

Answer: d. All of the above choices are good choices for patients with probable ACS except for glycoprotein IIb/IIIa inhibitor therapy, which carries a bleeding risk and may not improve the overall outcome of treatment.

Chapter 6: Head Trauma

This chapter covers the emergency medicine topic of head trauma. The head trauma patient may have a concussion or other minor injury and they may have either an open head injury (penetrating) or a closed head injury (blunt trauma). Injuries can also be very severe, resulting in severe brain contusions and intracerebral bleeding that can be life-threatening if not treated soon and aggressively.

Head Injury Definitions

There are several ways to define a head injury. A closed head injury is any head injury in which the patient receives blunt trauma or a sharp blow to the head that doesn't involve a penetrating injury and which can cause a variety of intracerebral or brain changes after the injury. An open or penetrating injury, by definition, involves a penetration into the skull that enters the brain cavity. This can be secondary to a gunshot wound, a knife wound, or a high-speed motor vehicle accident.

A concussion is defined as any injury which shakes the brain but doesn't cause any sort of internal bleeding. This is also called minimal brain injury and is the most likely result of a head injury. The actual definition of a "concussion" is any sudden or stunning, damaging, or shattering blow to the head, especially any jarring injury to the brain resulting in disturbance of cerebral function, usually a disturbance that is temporary.

A scalp wound is defined as any injury to the head that lacerates the skin overlying the brain. It generally doesn't result in an injury any deeper than the skin but causes significant bleeding because of the high degree of vascularity of the scalp area of the head. These generally require suturing or stapling in order to control the bleeding even though cosmesis is not usually necessary.

A skull fracture involves any breach in the bone, possibly secondary to a severe blow that breaks the bone or from a penetrating trauma that enters the bone, fracturing the bone and causing the brain cavity to be unprotected from external forces.

Bleeding inside the cranial vault can affect the meningeal layers outside of the brain. These include subdural hematomas (just beneath the dura mater), subarachnoid hemorrhages (beneath the arachnoid pia mater), and extradural hemorrhages (just outside the dura mater).

Intracerebral tissue bleeding involves any bleeding that affects the tissues of the brain itself. It is often accompanied by cerebral contusion and severe cognitive sequelae. The most severe injuries tend to cause Intracerebral bleeding and bruising.

Causes of Head injuries

- **Falls**—which can come from a great height or from a standing position.

- **Sports injuries**—which tend to be more common in patients who play contact sports.

- **Physical assaults**—which can result in a penetrating injury or blunt traumatic injury.

- **Traffic accidents**—particularly in cases where the patient wasn't buckled or protected with an airbag.

Symptoms of a Head Injury

There are a variety of symptoms of a head injury, which vary according to the severity of the injury. The symptoms can develop slowly over days or can occur suddenly with severe injuries. The head (on the outside) may appear normal; however, there could be symptoms from bleeding or swelling inside the skull. Secondary spinal cord injuries can occur from a primary head trauma.

Typical signs and symptoms of a concussion may include:

- Brief loss of consciousness

- Headache or a feeling of pressure in the head

- Periods of confusion or a "foggy feeling" in the head

- Amnesia of the event

- Dizziness or vertigo

- Nausea and vomiting

- Slurring of the speech, which is usually temporary

- Responding slowly to questions

- Feeling dazed shortly after the injury

- Tiredness

Signs that a concussion is severe and requires medical attention:

- Increasing rather than decreasing headache

- Seizures after the accident

- Inability to wake up after the accident

- Poor coordination or weakness

- Prolonged confusion

- Slurred speech

- Unequal pupil size

- Stiff neck

First Aid for Concussion

In treating the concussion patient, the first thing to do is to evaluate the person's ABCs or "airway, breathing, and circulation". If any of these are off or absent, CPR should begin per protocol. If two persons are present and who know CPR, then two-person CPR should be performed after 911 has been notified and are on their way.

If the ABCs are normal but the individual is unconscious, the spinal cord injury should be considered. This means stabilizing the neck and head—either manually or with a stiff cervical collar. No movement of the head should take place until EMS has arrived and has evaluated the patient.

Direct compression should be undertaken when a scalp laceration is present as they frequently bleed profusely. The only exception to this is the open skull fracture. In such cases, a sterile gauze should be placed over the wound with no attempt made to remove dirt or debris from the wound.

The vomiting patient should be rolled to the side in order to prevent aspiration. The head, neck, and body should be kept in alignment as much as possible if a cervical spine injury is present. A single episode of vomiting is common; however, multiple episodes of vomiting should be evaluated further by EMS services.

In areas of swelling, an ice pack should be provided to decrease the amount of swelling caused by external or internal bleeding of the head area. The wound should not be washed as this can exacerbate bleeding. Any object sticking out of a wound should be left in place. The person shouldn't be moved until EMS arrives. The person shouldn't be shaken and any helmet should be left on the patient if there is evidence of a serious head injury or cervical spine injury.

Subdural Hematoma

A subdural hematoma involves a bleeding inside the dura mater associates with a traumatic brain injury. The bleeding occurs beneath the dura mater but above the arachnoid mater. It usually comes from venous bleeding of vessels that bridge the two layers. The main complication of a subdural hematoma is increased intracranial pressure, which can damage the brain tissue. There are acute, subacute, or chronic subdural hematomas—of which acute subdural hematomas are the most severe and life-threatening.

Figure 10 shows a CT scan with a subdural hematoma:

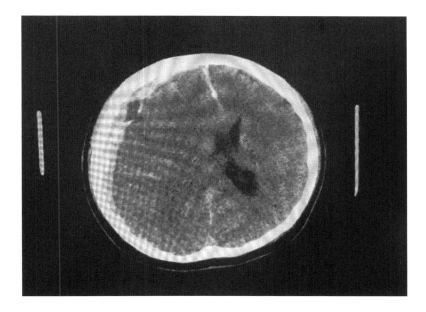

Figure 10

A subarachnoid hemorrhage is another type of intracranial hemorrhage, which results from bleeding between the arachnoid membrane and the pia mater around the brain. Finally, a person can have an epidural hematoma, which is very severe as it is caused by brisk bleeding resulting from tears of the arteries above the dura mater. This is the second most lethal type of intracranial hemorrhage and can lead to sudden death.

Figure 11 describes a CT scan showing a subarachnoid hemorrhage:

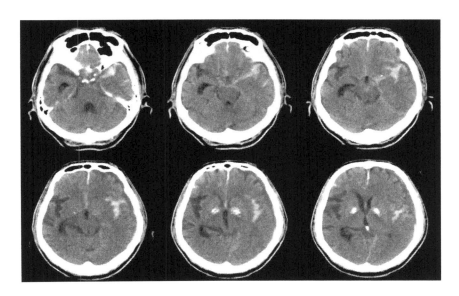

Figure 11

Acute subdural hematomas actually have the highest acute mortality rate as more force is necessary to create this type of injury and there is often diffuse brain injury coexisting with this hemorrhage type. The rate of mortality of subdural hematomas is about 80 percent. In chronic cases, half of all patients aren't identified for a few days or weeks as the head trauma is usually mild in nature. A few patients have a diagnosis that occurs years after the initial injury. The bleeding often stops spontaneously; however, rebleeding can happen. Chronic subdural hematomas are more common in elderly patients.

Signs and symptoms of a subdural hematoma can be sudden or build up over several hours or days. Chronic subdural hematomas may take as long as two weeks to develop. The main symptoms are secondary to an increased ICP (intracranial pressure). Typical signs and symptoms include a loss of consciousness, headache, seizure activity, amnesia, disorientation, nausea, vomiting, poor appetite, and changes in personality. Stroke-like symptoms include dysarthria, ataxia, altered breathing patterns, motor deficits, hearing loss, and abnormal eye movement.

Causes of Subdural Hematomas

These types of injuries rarely occur in the absence of a head injury that stretches and tears the bridging veins between the arachnoid layer and the dura mater layer. The subdural hematoma is much more common than epidural hemorrhages and results from shear forces in the brain. One classic injury in babies that results in a subdural hematoma is "shaken baby syndrome", which causes shear force when shaking a baby violently. Pre-retinal and retinal hemorrhages are a main finding seen in this type of injury. Patients on anticoagulants can have a subdural hemorrhage after a brief or minor trauma to the head.

Risk factors for a subdural hematoma include being very young or very old. The subdural space gets bigger with age so there is a greater likelihood of stress and friability of the bridging veins, which break easier than is the case with younger people. Babies also have a larger subdural space, making them greater candidates for having a subdural hematoma after being shaken. Other common risk factors include having dementia, having a cerebrospinal fluid leak, alcohol abuse, and being on blood thinning medications.

The most common cause of a traumatic brain injury is a motor vehicle accident, which accounts for 50% of all traumatic brain TBIs. Falls are the second leading cause of traumatic brain injury, accounting for 20 to 30% of all injuries to the brain. This is the leading cause of death in the very young and very old. Firearms are the third leading cause of traumatic brain injury, accounting for 12% of all TBI injuries. Nearly half of all brain injuries are work-related. Certain safety measures decrease the incidence of TBI. Alcohol use is also a risk factor for TBI.

Evaluating the Head Injury Patient

The definition of traumatic brain injury or TBI is any non-degenerative, non-congenital insult to the brain, usually from an externally-applied mechanical force that tends to lead to either temporary or permanent impairment of the person's psychosocial, physical, or cognitive functioning. A TBI is not exactly the same thing as a head injury as it implies an actual injury to brain tissue and not necessarily just an injury to the head itself.

The Glasgow Coma Scale or GCS defines just how severe a traumatic brain injury is when performed within 48 hours of the head trauma. There are several factors to the GCS, which are described:

- **Eye opening.** The patient is given 4 points for spontaneous eye opening, 3 points for opening the eyes to a voice, 2 points for opening the eyes to painful stimuli only, and one point for no response.

- **Motor response.** The patient is given 6 points for following commands, 5 points for localizing movements to pain, 4 points for withdrawing to pain, 3 points for decorticate (flexor) posturing, 2 points for decerebrate (extensor) posturing, and one point for no movement.

- **Verbal response.** The patient is given 5 points for being completely oriented, 4 points for being vocal but disoriented, 3 points for saying inappropriate words, 2 points for saying incomprehensible sounds, and 1 point for being non-verbal.

The range of points is 3-15. Scores of 3-8 indicate a severe TBI; a score of between 9 and 12 indicates a moderate TBI; a score of between 13 and 15 indicates a mild TBI.

The actual definition of a TBI (according to the American Congress of Rehabilitation Medicine includes the following criteria (only one is necessary to make the diagnosis):

- Loss of consciousness for any length of time

- Amnesia, either retrograde or anterograde

- Alteration in mental status at the time of the incident

- Focal neurological deficits (which can be permanent or transient)

Mild TBI can be defined by the following criteria:

- Having a GCS score of 13-15

- Having no CT scan findings of the brain

- Having a hospital stay of under two days

- Having no operative lesions

The following criteria are used to define moderate TBI:

- Length of hospital stay of at least 48 hours

- GCS score of 9-12

- The finding of an intracranial lesion

- Abnormal findings on CT scan

The following criteria are used to define severe TBI:

- A brain injury resulting in loss of consciousness of greater than 6 hours

- A Glasgow Coma Scale of 3 to 8

- Abnormal findings on CT scan

- Lengthy hospital stays

- Post-traumatic amnesia longer than 24 hours

There are four sub-classifications of severe TBI:

- Coma—unconsciousness that cannot be resolved by trying to awaken the patient; patient also remains unresponsive to noxious stimuli, has loss of a typical sleep-wake cycle, and is unable to engage in voluntary actions.

- Vegetative state—the patient is not comatose but is not aware of their environment

- Persistent vegetative state—being in a vegetative state for longer than one month

- Minimally responsive state—the patient interacts with the environment but still has impairment and inconsistency in their reactivity with the environment

It is difficult to identify the exact incidence and prevalence of TBI in the general public. Many mild cases are treated without having to see an emergency room doctor so they aren't reported. In addition, severe TBI patients may be dead before arriving to the hospital so they aren't reported either. CT scanning is the diagnostic tool of choice in evaluating TBI and it isn't done in every case, depending on the patient's symptoms. CT scanning has replaced plain films in identifying skull fractures.

Even with the limited ability to get the exact incidence of TBI, it has been shown that TBI accounts for approximately 40 percent of all deaths from injury in the U.S, with about 200,000 TBI victims requiring hospital visits. About 2 million people per year will have at least a mild traumatic brain injury. The total healthcare costs and other related costs, such as disability costs and the loss of income from a brain injury are very high. About 53,000 people die in the US as a result of a TBI.

The initial Glasgow Coma Scale score predicts the severity of the traumatic brain injury and predicts the likelihood of death from the injury. Mortality rate in severe TBI is about 33%, while the mortality rate in moderate TBI is about 2.5%.

Mortality rate of TBI is higher among children ages 0 to 4 years. The highest rate is found among black children who sustain a TBI motor vehicle accident between the ages of zero and nine years. About 2.5 to 6.5 million people in the US are currently living with disability related to having a previous TBI. About 1.9 million people will have a skull fracture per year. Mild TBI happens in approximately 130 cases out of 100,000 people.

People with the highest risk of having a TBI include the very young and very old, people of low socioeconomic status, single individuals, people in minority ethnic groups, being of the male gender, having a history of substance abuse, and having a previous TBI. Men have twice the risk of having of TBI, except for those who are elderly. Men have six times the risk of having a firearm -related TBI and twice the risk of having a motor vehicle-related TBI. TBI is the major cause of death related to injury in young people with peak incidence at 15 to 30 years of age. About 31 out of 100,000 elderly people die from a traumatic brain injury every year.

There are three mechanisms of injury in traumatic brain injury. The first of these is the collision of the head with a solid object at high speed. This is called impact loading. Another mechanism is called impulse loading, which involves sudden movement of the head without any impact. The third is called static loading and involves a head injury unrelated to a high-speed impact. Static loading is somewhat rare and involves the gradual squeezing of the skull.

Tissue injury can be of three types, including tissue compression, tissue stretching (tensile force), and shear forces resulting in tissue injury. Primary injuries can be focal, such as penetrating injuries, contusions, lacerations, hematomas within the skull, and skull fractures. They can also be diffuse, such as is seen in a diffuse axonal injury.

Skull Fractures

There are two types of skull fractures, including basilar skull fractures and fractures of the cranial vault. Typical complications can include cranial nerve damage, epidural or subdural hematoma, or internal brain damage. Fractures of the cranial vault can to be linear, and can be open or closed. Another way to define a fracture of the skull is to define them as depressed or nondepressed. Depressed skull fractures are more serious because they can put pressure on the brain. A simple fracture has just one bone fragment, while a compound fracture as at least two bony fragments.

Damage to the temporal region of the skull can cause hearing loss or vestibular dysfunction, even if there is no fracture. Conductive hearing loss usually involves an injury to the external or middle ear, while a sensorineural hearing loss involves damage to the inner ear or brain. If the crystals inside the ear become damaged, dizziness or vertigo can occur. The dizziness usually gets worse when there are sudden changes in head position.

Coup and Contrecoup Injuries

Coup and contracoup injuries are two different closed-head injuries. Both types of injuries are related to cerebral contusions. A primary coup injury occurs directly at the site of trauma because of pressure on the brain, while a contrecoup injury occurs on the opposite side of the direct impact. In some cases, the contrecoup injury is considered worse than the coup injury. Injuries over a large surface area are more likely to cause a contrecoup injury than injuries over a small surface area.

Diffuse Axonal Injury

This is the most diffuse type of injury that can happen in a closed head injury. In this type of injury, there is widespread, generalized brain damage, especially in the white matter of the brain. It is caused by the effects of high-speed acceleration and deceleration to the brain. It can also be caused by profound ischemia after a traumatic brain injury. There are several grades of this type of injury, including the following:

- **Grade 1**—this occurs when the axonal injury is mainly in the parasagittal white matter of the brain, particularly in the cerebral hemispheres.

- **Grade 2**—this includes the same lesions seen in grade 1 along with lesions of the corpus callosum.

- **Grade 3**—this includes the same lesions in grade 2 disease along with lesions of the cerebral peduncle.

Brain Imaging in Head Injury Cases

As mentioned, the preferred imaging modality for head injuries is a CT scan. This can be completed within five minutes and usually has no motion artifacts. It can find bleeding abnormalities including hematomas in the brain as well as skull fractures. It can be used when the patient is on life support. In actuality, magnetic resonance imaging or MRI is more sensitive and accurate for detecting contusions brain but is more time-consuming, more expensive, and can't be performed at all facilities. This type of scanning may not be compatible with life support and can't be used on all patients, particularly those of large size. CT scans may not show the injury until after 24 hours have gone by.

Skull radiography has limited use in detecting traumatic brain injuries. It can be used look for skull fractures but may not see a simple linear fracture that is not depressed. There is a high false negative rate for skull fracture using radiography, but there are few false positives. The CT scan has largely replaced this modality in detecting skull fractures.

Functional nuclear imaging is not widely used in traumatic brain injury assessment. On the other hand, the single photon emission computed tomography test or SPECT scan uses technetium 99m, is particularly sensitive at detecting decreased blood flow in areas of the brain affected by trauma. It is more sensitive than either CT scan or MRI scan, but it is expensive and may not be necessary in the detection of traumatic brain injury.

Positron emission tomography or PET scanning may or may not be helpful in traumatic brain injury cases. They take a long time to complete and cost approximately $2000 per test. They are also not available at most facilities, making them less useful in detecting traumatic brain injury.

Angiography can be helpful in TBI evaluation, as it can detect focal vascular spasms in the acute phase of the injury. This type of testing can detect traumatic aneurysms; however, these are quite rare, making the use of angiography something a clinician would do only if there was a great deal of suspicion that there might be a traumatic aneurysm. A conventional angiogram can be used to determine if there is a thrombus or active hemorrhaging, and in cases where the vascular lesions size is unknown.

CT scanning without contrast is the preferred diagnostic procedure in cases of subarachnoid hemorrhage and can be used along with angiography to find the site of the hemorrhage. The sensitivity of this procedure in detecting subarachnoid hemorrhage has increased so much that angiography is less likely to be performed.

The only time that MRI imaging is preferred over CT scanning is in cases of diffuse axonal injury. These types of injuries are extremely subtle and can often only be seen on MRI scans.

Head Injury Complications

The most serious complication of a head injury is brainstem herniation. This comes from increased intracranial pressure that pushes the brainstem through the foramen magnum, resulting in respiratory arrest and sudden death. Other types of herniation can involve an ipsilateral medial shift of the brain the other side, uncal herniation, which involves medial displacement of the uncus and the hippocampal gyrus, central transtentorial herniation, which involves downward displacement of the brain, and cerebellar herniation, which compresses the medulla, leading to both bradycardia and sudden death from respiratory arrest.

Another complication of traumatic brain injury is called chronic traumatic encephalopathy. This is seen in boxers and football players who sustain multiple traumatic injuries of the brain. The major findings are atrophy of multiple areas of the brain, ventricular dilation, and accumulation of the tau protein in the brain. These patients will have progressive dementia, anger episodes, episodes of aggression, and periods of depression. In fact, about 96% of football players played in the NFL was found to have evidence of chronic traumatic encephalopathy on autopsy in one study.

Other complications of a traumatic brain injury include posttraumatic seizures, deep vein thrombosis, hydrocephalus, spasticity, gastrointestinal complaints, urinary tract complaints, posttraumatic agitation, and gait abnormalities.

Treatment of Head Injuries in the Emergency Department

Because most head injuries are mild, little or no treatment is recommended. The workup can be primarily clinical observation and examination unless the injury is associated with being on blood thinners or is more severe than initially predicted. The only real treatment in the situation is to send the patient home with a head injury instruction sheet. Patients should be awakened every two hours and should return to the emergency department if symptoms don't gradually resolve over 24 hours.

Patients with moderate or severe head injuries may need stabilization to prevent hypoxia and hypotension. They need oxygen therapy and fluid resuscitation if necessary. Severely high oxygen concentrations have been associated with increased fatality so they don't need to be hyper-oxygenated. A CT scan is obtained after a complete neurological assessment. If patients have a large hematoma with a midline shift, a depressed skull fracture, or an open skull fracture need surgical intervention.

The head of the bed should be elevated if the patient is not hypotensive. Sedation has been found to be helpful in these patients. There is no evidence that anticonvulsants are helpful. Intracranial pressure monitoring is a good idea in serious cases, particularly if the GCS score is less than nine points. Hyperventilation has been found to reduce intracranial pressure in some cases. Although it also poses the risk of cerebral ischemia when hyperventilation is prolonged and thus should only be used as a short temporizing measure Mannitol is an osmotic diuretic that is most commonly used to decrease intracranial pressure in severely head-injured patients.

The traumatic brain injury patient with penetrating head trauma needs two components of treatment addressed. The first part of treatment is addressing increased intracranial pressure, which is common in high velocity missile injuries. The second part of the treatment involves removing the penetrating body and any devitalized tissue. These wounds are often dirty wounds with a high rate of infection if not treated appropriately.

Key Takeaways

- Head injuries can be mild concussions or severe traumatic brain injuries resulting in death.

- The CT scan is the imaging test of choice for traumatic brain injuries.

- Acute subdural hematoma has the highest risk of death among all intracranial hematomas.

- The treatment of severe head injuries involves respiratory support, oxygenation, elevating the head of the bed, and decreasing intracranial pressure.

Quiz

1. Which type of injury to the head results in the most severe neurological sequelae?

   a. Skull fracture

   b. Subdural hematoma

   c. Concussion

   d. Intracranial hemorrhage

Answer: d. The most severe neurological sequelae come from an intracranial hemorrhage, which involves bleeding inside the brain tissue itself.

2. What symptom would lead you to believe that that a head injury is more than just a concussion?

   a. Amnesia around the event

   b. Nausea and vomiting

   c. Hemiparesis

   d. Confusion

Answer: c. The main finding that would predict a worse prognosis and something worse than a mild concussion would be hemiparesis, which indicates a severe head injury.

3. You are evaluating a person with a severe head injury and possible concussion. What do you do first to evaluate the patient?

   a. Evaluate the airway

   b. Palpate the cervical spine

   c. Evaluate the pupil size

   d. Do a brief neurological examination

Answer: a. In any head injury case, the patient's airway should be evaluated and managed before any other evaluation.

4. You suspect a baby has shaken baby syndrome. What is the most common clinical finding in this case?

   a. Seizures

   b. Stiff neck

   c. Loss of consciousness

   d. Retinal hemorrhages

Answer: d. The most common clinical finding in a baby with shaken baby syndrome is retinal hemorrhages from increased intracranial pressure. The other findings are less likely to be found in this syndrome.

5. What is not considered a major risk factor for a subdural hematoma/hemorrhage?

    a. Being an infant

    b. Having dementia

    c. Being a smoker

    d. Being on warfarin

Answer: c. The above choices are all considered risk factors for a subdural hematoma except for being a smoker, which is not considered a risk factor.

6. What range of GCS scores indicate the presence of a severe TBI in a patient?

    a. 0-3

    b. 3-8

    c. 9-12

    d. 13-18

Answer: b. The range of scores for TBI is 3-15, with a score of 3-8 indicating a severe TBI injury.

7. What is the peak age of onset of TBI?

    a. 0-4 years

    b. 10-14 years

    c. 15-30 years

    d. 40-65 years

Answer: c. The peak age of onset of TBI in men and women is 15-30 years of age.

8. What is not considered a primary force in a closed head injury?

    a. Tensile force

    b. Shear force

    c. Compressive force

    d. Penetrating force.

Answer: d. All of the above are considered forces involved in a closed head injury except for a penetrating force, which is not seen in this type of injury.

9. Sensorineural hearing loss can occur in one of several ways. Which is not considered an area of damage likely to cause sensorineural hearing loss?

a. The eighth cranial nerve

b. The inner ear

c. The tympanic membrane

d. The temporal lobe

Answer: c. Damage to the temporal lobe, the eighth cranial nerve, or the inner ear and cause sensorineural hearing loss, however, damage to the tympanic membrane causes conductive hearing loss.

10. Which type of drug therapy is best used in the management of increased intracranial pressure in patients with traumatic head injury?

a. Furosemide

b. Corticosteroids

c. Spironolactone

d. Mannitol

Answer: d. Mannitol is an osmotic diuretic that is particularly useful in the management of increased intracranial pressure among patients with traumatic head injury.

Chapter 7: The Injured Eye

Injury is the most common reason for eye-related emergency department (ED) visits. The incidence of eye injuries requiring emergency department medical attention in the US is estimated to be between 500 and 1000 patients per 100,000 population. This chapter will cover some of the more common eye injuries seen in emergency medicine along with the treatment of these diseases.

Preventing Eye Injuries

Eye injuries can be prevented in many cases by wearing safety goggles. Patients often get an eye injury while using a lawn mower or leaf blower outside, using power tools like saws and drills, or working with metal-based machinery in the workplace. Ideally, safety goggles should wrap around the front, bottom, and sides of the eye in order to decrease the likelihood of having small, airborne particles penetrating the edges of the glasses. The best eyewear is made of polycarbonate lenses available from eye specialists.

Patients who wear prescription lenses should be offered prescription-strength safety glasses that either take the place of regular glasses or fit snuggly behind regular safety glasses. This is in complete compliance with OSHA recommendations. Patients have a higher risk of an eye injury in the workplace if they use certain power tools, are performing a new task, are working overtime, are in a hurry, are distracted, or feel tired at the time they are doing the task.

Air bags are a common source of eye injuries. Newer bags use less force than older bags so they are safer but still carry the risk of eye injuries as they deploy very fast and often deploy before the patient has a chance to close his or her eyes. The most common injury to the eye from an airbag is a corneal abrasion. The risk of this can be decreased by wearing a seatbelt, sitting far away from the steering wheel, and avoiding smoking while driving. Children should always sit in the back seat of the car as they have a higher risk of injury secondary to an airbag deployment.

Laser pointers are a preventable source of injury to the eye. These shine a high intensity, red light used in corporate and school presentations, as well as in the home as a toy. It can result in temporary blindness or even permanent retinal damage. Because of the danger, these devices come with warning labels indicating that the person shouldn't look into the light. The megawatt power is the determining factor in the degree of injury sustained by these devices. They are held to a legal limit of 5 megawatts but some people can get higher megawatt devices on the internet.

Urgent treatment of eye injuries can prevent permanent vision or eye loss. This highlights the importance of seeing the emergency medicine specialist or ophthalmologist to have the eye evaluated and treated. This is especially true for deep penetrating injuries from a work accident or accident in the home. Even corneal abrasions need to be seen in order to look for a foreign body and to prevent infections.

Corneal Abrasions

This involves a scratch on the cornea, which overlies the iris or the colored part of the eye. Having such a cause yields a persistent foreign body sensation, redness to the eye, and photophobia. The extent of the laceration which can be done with a fluorescein staining technique and the eye should be evaluated for a retained foreign body. Iron-containing scratches can have an imbedded foreign body with a rust ring that needs removal. This can be done using a powerful microscope that looks at the corneal structure and can visualize the rust ring. Bacterial and fungal infections can develop within 24 hours so medicated eye drops should be used. The eye should never be patched as this promotes bacterial overgrowth. Figure 12 shows a corneal abrasion seen on fluorescein staining:

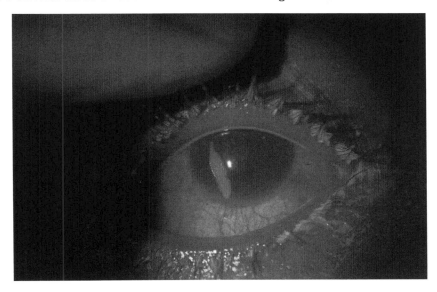

Figure 12

Penetrating Foreign Bodies in the Eye

These can involve metal projectiles or fish hooks that actually penetrate the globe. This is a medical emergency that requires urgent attention in the emergency room. Patients should be instructed to cover the eye with a paper cup and avoid removing the foreign body themselves. They shouldn't flush the eye or touch it in any way. Smaller foreign bodies cannot be seen but imbed into the cornea, giving symptoms much like a corneal abrasion. These types of foreign bodies and any rust rings should be urgently removed so as to prevent permanent infection and scarring of the eye. Surgery may be necessary with an ophthalmologist to remove the larger foreign bodies.

Chemical Burns of the Eye

The biggest problem with some workplaces is exposing the eye to an alkaline substance, an acidic substance or a solvent. Some of these substances will cause a burning or stinging sensation in the eye (but will be harmless), while others can cause serious injury to the eye. The two most dangerous things to get in the eye are acidic substances and alkaline substances, with alkaline substances being the more damaging of the two. Alkaline substances cause caustic destruction of the external eye tissue and can result in vision loss. Acidic substances will also cause possible damage to the eye but to a lesser degree. Solvents are irritating but tend not to cause permanent damage to the eye.

Acidic substances will burn the eye but are easily washed out, leaving little in the way of permanent scarring or eye damage. Exposure to alkaline substance is much more serious but doesn't result in as much eye pain or redness. Toilet bowel cleaners, oven cleaners, and chalk dust can cause alkaline injuries to the eye. They can get in the eye by a splash injury or by rubbing the eye with an alkaline or acidic substance.

60

The main treatment for any type of splash injury is to apply a stream of lukewarm water over the eye surface for about fifteen minutes using a faucet. Then call the emergency room or eye doctor for further instructions. If the vision is blurry and the eye is red, the patient should go to the emergency department for further evaluation. A cool compress can be placed over the eye but no rubbing of the eye surface should take place. Depending on what caused the problem, there may be only minor eye irritation or permanent blindness.

Eye Contusions

There can be ecchymosis of the eyelid, swollen eyelids, and eye pain from being struck by an object directly into the eye itself. This is commonly called "a black eye". The treatment of choice for this is an ice pack to reduce swelling and decrease bleeding of the soft tissues. These injuries should be evaluated so that the eye can be assessed for any additional injury.

Subconjunctival Hemorrhages

This presents as a bright red eye in the white part of the eye that looks really dramatic but is completely harmless. It can come from rubbing the eye, sneezing, minor trauma, or coughing causing breakage of the blood vessels beneath the conjunctiva of the eye. There are no visual deficits and the eye is only red over the white part of the eye. The entire sclera can be red. These often don't hurt at all and don't affect vision. There are no treatments for this condition and it resolves spontaneously over about 7-10 days.

Traumatic Iritis

This involves an inflammation of the colored portion of the eye surrounding the pupil. It is often secondary to a blunt traumatic injury to the eye, which may be minor. It causes pain and photophobia and needs treatment as there is a risk of permanent eye damage. The treatment of choice includes giving mydriatics that widen the pupil as much as possible, which allows the iris to rest. Steroid eyedrops are used to reduce inflammation of the eye, which can promote healing and improve the chances of a return to normal vision. Oral or injected corticosteroids are used if the drops alone don't resolve the issue.

Hyphemas

A hyphema is a serious eye injury stemming from blunt trauma to the eye. It causes bleeding in the anterior chamber of the eye (between the cornea and the iris). It causes a crescent of blood visible in the dependent part of the eye and reduced vision. The main treatment is rest and elevation of the head of the bed. NSAIDs, aspirin, and anticoagulants should be avoided. The eye is monitored for resolution of the bleeding. Sometimes 1 percent atropine is used to decrease the pressure on the eye. Anything that lowers the pressure of the eye is recommended. Sometimes beta blockers are used to prevent bleeding from high pressures in the eye.

Figure 13 shows what a hyphema looks like:

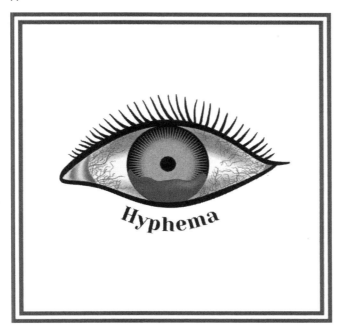

Figure 13

Blowout Fractures

This is a serious injury that stems from a significant blow to the eye. The pressure from a blowout injury causes a fracture to the facial bones that lead to the maxillary sinuses. It can cause a trapping of the external ocular muscles in the fracture site so that there is double vision when trying to look upward. If this occurs, there may need to be surgical intervention to free up the trapped muscle.

Signs of a Serious Eye Injury

Signs and symptoms of a possible serious eye injury include the following:

- An obvious laceration of the eyelid.

- Difficulty seeing out of the affected eye.

- Extreme pain in the affected eye.

- Lack of movement of the affected eye.

- Irregularity of the pupil or abnormal pupil size.

- Blood in the anterior chamber of the eye.

- Foreign body in the eye or persistent foreign body sensation in the eye.

As with any eye injury, the patient should be advised not to put pressure on the eye or rub the eye. The foreign body should never be removed except in the surgical suite or in the emergency department. No drops or ointment should be used by the patient. A possible severe eye injury should be seen urgently by the emergency room doctor or a qualified ophthalmologist.

If a cup is available, it should be taped over the eye to shield it. The eye should never be rinsed if punctured and no NSAIDS or aspirin should be given for pain control as this will enhance the risk of bleeding. Chemical burns should be flushed immediately with plain, clean water from the faucet before seeking medical attention in the emergency department.

If the patient has a black eye, they should be instructed to place a cool pack over the eye and to present for urgent evaluation of the eye. No pressure should be applied when the ice pack is placed on the eye. Any visual disturbance should be seen urgently. Sand or minor debris in the eye can be initially managed at home by flushing the eye. If a consistent foreign body sensation is noted, the patient needs to be evaluated for a retained foreign body, rust ring, or corneal abrasion.

Sudden Vision Loss in the ED

Sudden vision loss can occur over a few minutes or over a few days. It can affect a part of the visual field and can affect either one or both eyes. It may be seen as blurry vision or as a complete loss of vision. Sudden vision loss has three possible causes:

- Opacification of the lens, cornea, or vitreous part of the eye

- Injuries or damage to the retina

- Optic nerve or another visual pathway disruption

The most common cause of loss of vision is a vascular occlusion of the retinal vessels, such as a central retinal artery occlusion or a central retinal vein occlusion. Other possible causes include ischemic optic neuropathy (from temporal arteritis), vitreous hemorrhage (as is seen by diabetics in diabetic retinopathy) or traumatic injury to the eye.

Some eye disorders cause complete loss of vision in the affected eye, while things like a detached retina may affect only a portion of the visual field. An occlusion of a branch of the retinal artery or vein may cause partial vision loss.

Anterior uveitis can cause vision loss but usually causes severe eye pain so the patient presents for treatment before the vision is lost. Certain drugs can cause sudden vision loss (such as quinine, ergot alkaloids, salicylates, and methanol), and aggressive retinitis.

Amaurosis fugax causes blindness lasting a few minutes to a few hours and is secondary to cerebrovascular disease. A carotid ultrasound, echocardiogram, CT scan of the head, MRI scan of the head, and ECG should be done for patients who have suspected cerebrovascular disease as a cause of blindness without eye pain.

Temporal arteritis or giant cell arteritis will lead to loss of vision without eye pain. Sometimes headache, jaw pain, or tongue pain can suggest ischemia of the side of the head affected by the temporal artery. A tender temporal artery can suggest the diagnosis as can a high ESR, high C-reactive protein level, high platelet count, or positive findings in a temporal artery biopsy.

Macular hemorrhage can cause painless loss of vision secondary to neovascularization in patients with age-related macular degeneration. In this condition, there is blood to be found around the macula and deep to the retina that can be seen with clinical evaluation.

Nonarteritic ischemic optic neuropathy will show up with vision loss, optic disk edema, hemorrhages, and a past history of hypotension, hypertension, or diabetes. A temporal artery biopsy is needed to rule out temporal arteritis but will be negative.

An ocular migraine will have complete loss of vision, scintillating scotomata, or mosaic patterns in the vision that is followed by a typical migraine. It is seen in young people and is purely a clinical evaluation.

A retinal artery occlusion will be painless and sudden. The retina will be pale with a cherry-red fovea. Sometimes the site of the occlusion can be seen and the patient will have risk factors for heart disease and blood vessel disease. Tests for giant cell arteritis need to be performed as well as a carotid ultrasound, MRI scan of the head, CT scan of the head, ECG, and echocardiogram.

Retinal detachment is painless and is a clinical diagnosis. The patient will experience flashing lights and floaters in their recent history. There will be a visual field defect, advancing age, eye surgery, or recent trauma to suggest a risk for the detachment.

A retinal vein occlusion will be painless. There will be retinal hemorrhages and risk factors for hyperviscosity, diabetes, and/or hypertension. This is purely a clinical evaluation that can be seen on fundoscopy.

A transient ischemic attack or stroke will yield painless vision loss. The patient will have bilaterally symmetric visual field deficits and may have abnormalities on their echocardiogram or carotid ultrasound. Risk factors for stroke will be present.

There are numerous causes of loss of vision with eye pain, which can be distinguished from painless causes of eye vision loss. The most common is acute angle-closure glaucoma. There will be headache, halos around lights, nausea, red eye, corneal edema, a shallow anterior chamber and a high intraocular pressure. It can be seen clinically and a gonioscopy evaluation will clinch the diagnosis.

A corneal ulceration will cause a painful loss of vision. The ulcer can be seen on fluorescein staining with the naked eye or with a slit-lamp (microscopic) evaluation. Treating the painful ulcer will restore vision. This is often caused by excessive contact lens use.

Endophthalmitis is a painful loss of vision associated with conjunctival injection, decreased red reflex, and floaters in the eye. Cultures of the eye can show an organism causing the infection. Risk factors include having a previous ruptured globe, recent eye surgery, or an intraocular foreign body.

Optic neuritis may or may not have eye pain associated with loss of vision, which is usually central vision loss. There is pain with eye movement and a defect in the pupillary reflex (which is hyperreflexive). Color vision is impaired and an examination of the eye will show optic disk edema.

In evaluating the patient with sudden vision loss, the visual acuity should be measured. Visual field determination should be undertaken and documented. Light reflexes should be assessed as well as ocular motility. Color vision plates should assess he color vision and the cornea/sclera/conjunctiva should be assessed with a slit lamp and fluorescein staining. The lens should be evaluated for the presence of cataracts and the IOP should be measured. The pupil should be dilated with phenylephrine and/or cyclopentolate. After full dilation, the entire fundus should be thoroughly examined.

The specific pattern of vision loss gives the best way of determining the cause of the loss. If the red reflex is unable to be seen, this suggests opacification as a cause of vision loss. Retinal abnormalities can be seen when dilating the eye and looking at the retina. Detachment, retinal vein occlusion, and retinal artery occlusion will be relatively obvious on fundoscopy examination. If there is an absent direct pupillary light reflex but a normal consensual reflex, there is probably an abnormality of the retina or optic nerve.

Unilateral vision loss suggests a problem in front of the optic chiasm, while bilateral visual field deficits suggest a lesion behind the optic chiasm. Constant eye pain is most likely seen with a corneal ulcer, anterior chamber inflammation, or increased intraocular pressure. Temporal headaches indicate the possibility of temporal arteritis or an ocular migraine.

In some cases, there is optic neuritis from multiple sclerosis as the only finding in the disease. In order to determine if MS is the cause of the problem, a gadolinium-enhanced MRI can be done to make the diagnosis of MS as a cause of vision loss secondary to optic neuritis.

Key Takeaways

- The injured eye can involve a simple case of subconjunctival hemorrhage to a severe globe penetrating injury.

- Most eye injuries can be better treated if seen acutely in the emergency department or by an ophthalmologist.

- Patients shouldn't rub or patch an injured eye but should cover it with a plastic or paper cup taped to the face and present to the emergency room.

- There are painless causes of loss of vision as well as painful causes of loss of vision, which can effectively help in making the diagnosis of what is causing the vision loss.

Quiz

1. What is not considered a risk factor for an eye injury in the workplace?

    a. Wearing prescription goggles

    b. Being distracted on the job

    c. Doing an unfamiliar task

    d. Working with metallic machinery

Answer: a. All of the above put the patient at risk for developing an eye injury in the workplace except for wearing prescription goggles, which doesn't increase the risk of an eye injury.

2. What is the most common eye injury that can be sustained from an airbag deployment?

    a. Ruptured globe

    b. Hyphema

    c. Retinal detachment

    d. Corneal abrasion

Answer: d. The corneal abrasion is the most common type of eye injury that can happen in cases of an airbag deployment because the patient doesn't have time to close their eyes when the airbag deploys.

3. What is the legal limit for wattage in a laser light device?

    a. 1 megawatt

    b. 5 megawatts

    c. 20 megawatts

    d. 50 megawatts

Answer: b. The legal limit for wattage in a laser light device in the US is 5 megawatts. Even at this low wattage, there are warning labels on all devices to prevent people from staring into them.

4. What is the treatment of choice for an eye contusion?

    a. Flushing the eye with cool water

    b. Covering the eye with a patch for 24 hours

    c. Applying an ice pack to the effected eye

    d. Using saline eye drops to keep the eye surface moist

Answer: c. An ice pack to the affected eye will decrease swelling and will decrease bleeding in the affected eye and is the treatment of choice for an eye contusion.

5. What is the main treatment for a subconjunctival hemorrhage?

    a. Patching the eye for 24 hours

    b. Using topical pain drops to control pain

    c. Flushing the eye with cool water every 3-4 hours

    d. No treatment is recommended

Answer: d. There is no treatment recommended for patients who have a subconjunctival hemorrhage except for watchful waiting so that it can resolve in 7-10 days.

6. Which type of treatment is most helpful in reducing the pathology behind traumatic iritis?

    a. Steroid eye drops

    b. Antibiotic eye drops

    c. Mydriatic eye drops

    d. Antihistamine eye drops

Answer: a. Steroid eye drops can decrease inflammation, making it the greatest treatment choice in managing the underlying pathophysiology behind traumatic iritis.

7. What would be considered the main cause of sudden vision loss?

a. Trauma to the eye

b. Diabetic retinopathy

c. Central retinal artery occlusion

d. Temporal arteritis

Answer: c. The main cause of sudden vision loss would be central retinal artery occlusion, with the other causes being secondary or less common.

8. Which cause of vision loss can be identified by an elevated C-reactive protein level

a. Giant cell arteritis

b. Amaurosis fugax

c. Functional vision loss

d. Age-related macular degeneration

Answer: a. Giant cell arteritis can be identified by having an elevated C-reactive protein level.

9. Which of the following is not considered a painless acute loss of vision?

a. Giant cell arteritis

b. Narrow angle glaucoma

c. Retinal artery occlusion

d. Retinal detachment

Answer: b. Narrow angle glaucoma will have a sudden loss of vision associated with pain in the eye, which distinguishes it from the many painless causes of loss of vision.

10. Which cause of vision loss can be effectively evaluated by doing a gadolinium-enhanced MRI scan of the head?

a. Amaurosis fugax

b. Optic neuritis

c. Open-angle glaucoma

d. Central retinal occlusion

Answer: b. Otic neuritis can be secondary to multiple sclerosis so a gadolinium-enhanced MRI scan can evaluate this possibility.

Chapter 8: Chest Trauma

Chest trauma can occur secondary to many different things, including penetrating injuries, falls, and motor vehicle accidents. The different things that can cause chest trauma can affect the heart or the lungs, leading to cardiorespiratory compromise. This chapter will cover both blunt traumatic injuries of the chest and penetrating injuries of the chest and their implications.

Basic Anatomy and Background of Chest Trauma

Trauma of any kind is the leading cause of morbidity, hospitalization, death, and disability from the ages of one to fifty years of age. It is a major health problem that is somewhat preventable. Chest trauma is particularly prone to morbidity and mortality as it affects the heart and lungs—two primary structures in the chest. Blunt chest trauma can affect the bony skeleton (including the sternum, scapulae, clavicles, and ribs), the pleural lining and lungs, the trachea and bronchial tree, the heart, the esophagus, the great vessels around the heart, and the diaphragm.

Tests used to treat patients with chest trauma starts with an ultrasound (the FAST examination is often used), which can look for a hemothorax, cardiac tamponade, and other bleeding in the chest, CT scan of the chest (to look at the main vessel structures), endovascular techniques (to repair great-vessel damage), and both surgical and nonsurgical exploration when a treatable disease is found. Thoracoscopy can be done for high risk patient suspected of having a mediastinal injury.

The border of the thorax Is the thoracic inlet superiorly, just above the clavicles. This is where the major vessels enter and leave the heart. The thoracic outlet is the main outlet on the upper lateral part of the thorax. This sends and receives blood vessels to and from the upper extremities. The nerves form a plexus in the axillary area. The most important vein in this outlet is the subclavian vein. Inferiorly, the border of the thorax is the diaphragm. This allows the inferior vessels to exit the chest cavity into the abdomen.

There are muscles, bony ribs, rib cartilage, sternum, scapulae, and clavicles that make up the chest all. This the outer border to the chest cavity. There is an intercostal nerve, artery, and vein that supplies each rib and chest wall tissue. The parietal pleura lines the chest wall, while the visceral pleura lines the lungs themselves. The pericardium lines the heart. The lungs make up most of the thorax. There are two lungs, with the left lung having two lobes and the right lung having three lobes.

The heart is in the middle of the chest and received blood from the superior vena cava and the inferior vena cava. There are pulmonary vessels that send blood to the lungs and receives blood from the lungs via the pulmonary vein and pulmonary artery. Blood is oxygenated in the lungs at the level of the alveoli. The left ventricle of the heart sends oxygenated blood out of the aorta and into the circulation. The thoracic duct starts in the abdomen and rises through the thorax to enter into the subclavian vein.

The two thing that affect the chest in blunt trauma include some type of derangement of the airflow and oxygenation, or a derangement of the blood. Sepsis is much less common but can be caused by rupture of the esophagus, causing bacteria to enter the bloodstream. Rib fractures are common chest wall injuries, which can make breathing difficult. Direct contusions of the lungs are frequently linked to major chest blunt trauma. This creates shunting and dead-space ventilation, which causes the hypoxia seen in blunt trauma.

Other things that lead to oxygenation failure include hemothorax, pneumothorax, hemopneumothorax. They compress normal lung tissue, blocking it ability to oxygenate. The tension pneumothorax is the most severe of the chest wall traumas affecting the lungs as it compresses on the opposite side of the lungs.

After chest trauma, several mediators are released into the bloodstream. These include prostanoids, tissue necrosis factor (TNF), and interleukin-6 (IL-6), which bring about secondary changes to the lung and the heart. When serious cardiac injuries happen, the patient often dies for being seen or evaluated. They exsanguinate or suffer from severe heart pump failure, resulting in cardiogenic shock, hypovolemic shock, and death.

Causes and Epidemiology of Chest Trauma

The vast majority of chest trauma cases are secondary to motor vehicle accidents or MVAs, which account for up to 80% of blunt trauma injuries to the chest. Other types of injuries include assaults, falls, and pedestrian accidents. Blast injuries in wartime situations are also causes of blunt chest trauma. About 100,000 people die in the US from trauma with about 12 people out of 1 million having chest trauma. A third of these cases need urgent hospitalization. About one fourth of all trauma deaths are secondary to direct chest trauma. Only about 20% of cases are serious enough to require surgical intervention so the prognosis is excellent. Damage to the heart and great vessels carries a poorer prognosis.

Most blunt trauma patients can be treated with supportive therapy; however, 8% of cases need some kind of surgery. Immediate surgery is necessary for any injury that disrupts the chest wall integrity and for any blunt diaphragm injury. A massive air leak needs urgent intervention and surgery is required for any injury resulting in a hemothorax that doesn't get better with a chest tube. If there are gastrointestinal contents in the chest tube, urgent surgery is required. Late surgery is necessary to drain and empyema, traumatic lung abscess, or chronic hemothorax. A persistent thoracic duct fistula or a tracheoesophageal fistula will require late surgery.

Urgent reasons to have surgery with an injury to the heart or great vessels include having a cardiac tamponade, great vessel injury on radiographic testing, or pulmonary embolism. If a great vessel injury identified soon, it may be a reason for later surgery.

Rib Fractures

The most common injury seen in blunt thoracic trauma is a rib fracture. The fourth through 10th ribs are those that are more frequently involved in fracture. Patients complain of chest pain is reproducible to palpation. There can be crepitus over the site of the fracture and evidence of pneumothorax with decreased breath sounds overlying the fracture. Rib fractures aren't always benign and can indicate a more severe internal chest injury. About 50% of patients with cardiac injury have at least one rib fracture. Fractures of the eighth through 12th ribs may indicate abdominal injury, particularly of the liver. Older patients with at least three rib fractures have a fivefold increase in mortality and a fourfold increase in pneumonia.

Figure 14 shows rib fractures on chest x-ray:

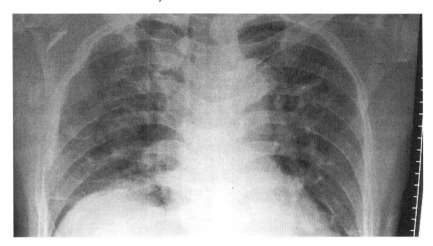

Figure 14

The main treatment for rib fractures is pain control. This can involve oral pain control or parenteral pain control. Some patients do well with intercostal nerve blocks or local anesthetic injected directly into the area of the fracture. Bupivacaine the most common local anesthetic used. Patients with multiple rib fractures can do well with an epidural anesthetic. Early ambulation will speed healing. Surgery is almost never required. Complications include flail chest and nonunion.

Flail Chest

Flail chest involves having three or more rib fractures locate next to one another, which allows for a free-floating, unstable chest wall segment. It can also be caused by a dislocation the ribs from the cartilage. There will be localized pain that worsens on inspiration and shortness of breath. The chest wall fragment sinks in with inspiration and pouches outward with expiration. The patient may tire from this type off ineffective breathing. Associated injuries are common as these are generally high-impact lesions. This makes the rate of mortality high in cases of flail chest. The treatment of choice for severe cases in intubation and mild fluid resuscitation as they can develop respiratory congestion and pulmonary edema. Surgical fixation is the definitive treatment of choice for these patients.

First and Second Rib Fractures

The fractures to the first and second ribs involve much more energy than is seen in other rib fractures and these are more dangerous because of the underlying injuries seen in these types of fractures. Fractures to these areas involve major head injuries, major thoracic injuries, major vascular injuries, and concomitant abdominal injuries. If these types of fractures are found, they are rarely isolated and require the exclusion of other injuries at the same time. The main treatment is pain control and the treatment of other injuries.

Clavicle Fractures

These are the most common injuries seen in shoulder injuries of the chest area. It happens with a fall on an outstretched hand or a direct blow to the clavicle. About 80 percent happen in the midportion of the clavicle. There is tenderness and sometimes a deformity of the clavicle with reproducibility of the pain upon palpating the clavicle. The proximal part of the clavicle is displaced superiorly because of the attachment to the sternocleidomastoid muscle. Almost all can be treated with a figure-of-eight dressing, a sling, or a clavicle strap. Rarely is surgery necessary unless the fracture is severely displaced.

Sternoclavicular Joint Dislocations

These involve a dislocation secondary to an extreme lateral compressive force against the shoulder. Anterior dislocations are more common than posterior dislocations. Patients will have arm pain and displacement of the shoulder. The medial end of the clavicle can be more prominent on the affected side. Associated injuries include the trachea, brachial plexus, or subclavian vessels—mainly seen in posterior dislocations. The treatment of choice is the application of local anesthesia and the use of sedation before relocating the dislocation. In some cases, general anesthesia is necessary for closed reduction. If this fails, an open reduction procedure may be necessary.

Sternal Fractures

The vast majority of sternal fractures take place secondary to motor vehicle accidents. Usually the upper and middle third of the bones are affected. The main symptom is reproducible pain in the sternum with localized swelling and tenderness. There may be bruising to the anterior chest wall. Up to 70% of patients will have underlying internal injuries. The most common other injuries include closed head injuries, rib fractures, and long bone fractures. Fewer than 20% of patients will have a blunt cardiac contusion. Even so, an ECG should be obtained. There is generally no treatment for this type of injury other than pain control and rest. The treatment of underlying injuries can also be undertaken.

Scapular Fractures

Scapular fractures are not very common. The main reason they are important is that a high-energy force is required so that there is a high incidence of other injuries. Up to 100% of the time, there is some other injury such as an injury to the head, abdomen, or chest. The pain is localized around the scapula with bruising and swelling being common features. Usually the body or neck of the scapula is fractured. These can be easily missed as they are difficult to find on chest x-ray. If they are found, a thorough evaluation for secondary injuries should be performed. The treatment of choice is shoulder immobilization with early range of motion exercises. Surgical treatment is rare.

Scapulothoracic Dissociation

Patients with flail shoulder, which is also called scapulothoracic dissociation, involves a disruption of the shoulder-girdle so that the scapula is pulled away from the chest wall. There can be a significant hematoma and swelling of the affected area as well as neurological deficit to the affected arm and shoulder. Surgery is rarely indicated as an emergency surgery unless there is significant disruption of the neurovascular bundles. Severe and permanent disability can result from this, including having to have an above the elbow amputation.

Soft Tissue Chest Wall Injuries

Large chest wall open injuries involve irrigation of the wound and debridement of nonviable tissue. This is the best way to prevent a necrotizing wound infection. Large injuries may require skin grafting or other reconstructive surgery to restore the integrity of the chest wall.

Traumatic Asphyxia

This is a clinical syndrome that occurs after a severe crushing injury to the chest, especially one in which the patient is pinned under a large object for a long period of time. The presenting complaint is cyanosis of the head and neck, ecchymosis around the eyes, conjunctival hemorrhage, and petechiae of the head and neck. It can be so severe that the patient has loss of consciousness, temporary blindness, or seizures. It stems from closure of the glottis during the crush injury. There are often significant traumatic injuries to the torso and head, many of which need to be treated surgically.

Blunt Traumatic Injuries to the Diaphragm

Diaphragm injuries are relatively uncommon with blunt chest trauma. If they do occur, they are usually secondary to a motor vehicle accident at high speeds. These cause about a third of all diaphragmatic injuries. They can occur on either side of the diaphragm and can cause abdominal injuries or chest injuries. Hypovolemic shock is a common finding because of major splenic and liver injuries. Usually the plain film x-ray is normal unless the stomach has risen into the chest cavity. The CT scan is not accurate enough and the MRI scan is not available at most facilities. The imaging test of choice is therefore an ultrasound of the chest and abdomen. Diagnostic laparoscopy and diagnostic thoracoscopy are also good ways of determining diaphragmatic injuries.

As these tears tend to be 5 to 10 cm or longer, surgery is the best choice for treatment. Most patients need a laparotomy as this also look for other injuries. A chest approach can also be helpful in repairing these types of injuries. Injuries that can be repaired primarily can be repaired using synthetic mesh as polypropylene mesh or mesh made from Dacron.

Pneumothorax

The main cause of a pneumothorax in blunt chest trauma occurs when a fractured rib enters the lung parenchyma. They can also result from a deceleration injury or from barotrauma to the lung is unassociated with any type of rib fracture. Rarely direct injuries to the lungs will cause a pneumothorax. There will be sharp pain on inspiration and pain on palpation of the rib fractures. There will be decreased breath sounds over the area affected and a hemothorax is extremely common. These patients require pain control and a chest tube in order to get rid of the blood and air in the space outside of the lungs.

Figure 15 shows a pneumothorax on chest x-ray:

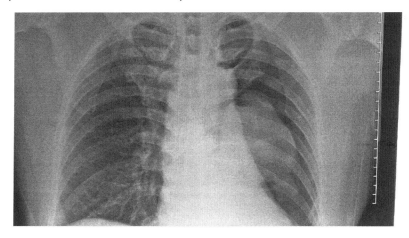

Figure 15

An open pneumothorax can occur with either a blunt trauma to the chest or a penetrating trauma to the chest. These patients have extreme shortness of breath and an obvious chest wall defect. There are loss of breath sounds on the affected area and a possibility of hemodynamic instability if a tension pneumothorax develops. The treatment of choice is to apply an occlusive dressing over the wound and to give a chest tube in order to drain the air and blood from the chest cavity. They often need operative management with debridement of the wound and closure of the defect.

Tension Pneumothorax

The same types of trauma that produce a regular pneumothorax can produce a tension pneumothorax. The major difference is that there is ongoing leakage of air from the lung parenchyma increasing the amount of air outside of the lungs and increasing the pressure outside of the lungs. These patients have marked respiratory distress, decreased breath sounds over the pneumothorax site, deviation of the trachea, and sometimes cardiovascular collapse. The treatment of choice is to insert a large-bore needle in the second intercostal space relieve the tension followed by a tube thoracostomy procedure. Figure 16 shows a tension pneumothorax on x-ray:

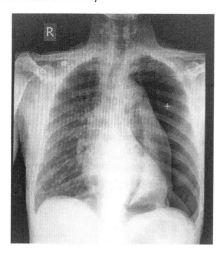

Figure 16

Hemothorax

A hemothorax involves a buildup of blood in the pleural space from some type of bleeding that can be either in the chest wall, a major intrathoracic vessel, or from the lung parenchyma. These patients are short of breath and will have chest pain on the side of their injury. There will be decreased breath sounds over the hemothorax. The main treatment is to evacuate the hemothorax by placing a chest tube on the side of the injury. Sometimes several chest tubes need to be placed. Surgery is reserved for those cases that do not resolve spontaneously after chest tube placement. Hemothoraces that have clotted may result in the need for surgery to evacuate the clot in order to prevent infection and fibrothorax.

Figure 17 is a hemothorax on chest x-ray:

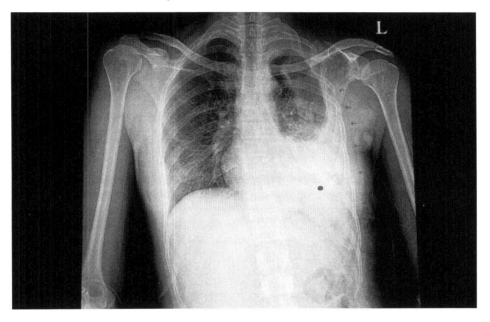

Figure 17

Pulmonary Contusions

High forces to the chest can result in a pulmonary contusion. The main finding is an infiltrate in the lungs with hemorrhaging into the lung tissue. Patients will have respiratory distress and decreased breath sounds over the affected area. Overlying fractured ribs are not uncommon. The treatment is pain control, supplemental oxygen, and possible intubation if the patient is having respiratory distress. Rarely surgery, including a pneumonectomy may need to be performed; however, this surgery carries a mortality rate greater than 50%.

Tracheal Injuries

Blunt trauma can affect the trachea as well; however, the risk is as low as 1%. The mortality rate is extremely high, with most patients dying in route to the hospital. There are usually many other coexisting injuries with this type of trauma. The mechanism of injury is a sudden compression of the trachea or a deceleration injury. Patients who survive are in severe respiratory distress and cannot talk. Inspiratory and expiratory stridor are common and many patients also have a pneumothorax. There is often a massive amount of subcutaneous air, which clinches the diagnosis. These are life-threatening injuries that require immediate bronchoscopy and surgical repair. These patients need endotracheal intubation preferably under bronchoscopic guidance. The end of the tube must be passed below the level of the injury.

Blunt Bronchial Injuries

Blunt bronchial injuries happen because of severe deceleration, such as is seen in a high impact motor vehicle accident. Most of these patients die of ventilatory failure before they can be adequately treated. The signs and symptoms include respiratory distress and a huge pneumothorax. Breath sounds are extremely diminished on the affected side and there may be subcutaneous air. Tension pneumothorax is possible and there can be massive blood loss from related injuries. This is an extremely life-threatening injury.

Blunt Esophageal Injuries

Esophageal injuries are rare because of the esophagus as well protected behind the trachea. They are caused by an increase in intraluminal pressure of the esophagus after blunt trauma to the chest. Most occur in the cervical area and there are often other organs damaged. Subcutaneous air and free air in the abdomen are typical findings. Patients who are not detected early enough will have systemic sepsis. The treatment of choice is IV antibiotics against gram-positive organisms and anaerobes. Surgical correction is necessary with the placement of chest tubes to drain any abscesses or bleeding.

Blunt Pericardial Injuries

It is rare to have a blunt pericardial injury as most of these injuries are penetrating injuries. The biggest risk is herniation of the heart outside of the pericardial sac, which results in decreased cardiac output. A pericardial rub may be heard on auscultation. If these defects are large enough, they need to be repaired surgically, sometimes using a patch or graft to repair large defects.

Blunt Cardiac Injuries

Motor vehicle accidents are the most common reason behind a blunt cardiac injury. The injury can be a minor injury or a severe injury involving rupture of valves, the myocardium, or the interventricular septum. Most patients do not require any type of treatment; however, some patients will have severe cardiac tamponade and complete cardiovascular collapse, from a loss of ability to pump blood around the body. Arrhythmias can be treated with antiarrhythmic drugs and severe injuries may require surgery, particularly those with a cardiac rupture (if they survive the trip to surgery). Rapid pericardiocentesis will help patients with cardiac tamponade. This can be done in the emergency department without the need for emergency surgery.

Another blunt trauma issue related to the heart is called commotio cordis or sudden cardiac death in a healthy individual thing some type of sport that causes a direct blow to the heart. The blow causes ventricular fibrillation that is sudden in onset. Rapid CPR and defibrillation can save these patients if they are started within minutes of the cardiac arrest.

Blunt Injuries to the Thoracic Aorta and other Major Arteries

The most common cause of a blunt injury to the thoracic aorta is a high-speed motor vehicle accident, with less common causes being a fall or a pedestrian accident. The injury usually comes as a result of rapid deceleration and compression at certain points in the artery. Many of these people die at the scene from exsanguination before reaching the emergency department. This makes these types of injuries else common cause of death besides head injuries in a motor vehicle accident. The treatment of choice is lowering the blood pressure as much as possible with beta blockers until definitive surgery can be performed.

Blunt Injuries to Superior Vena Cava

Injuries to the superior vena cava and other major veins in the thorax are not common. The mechanism of injury is similar to that of the aorta, with deceleration being the major factor behind this type of injury. The treatment of choice is called a lateral venorrhaphy, which involves surgical repair of the disrupted vein.

Penetrating Thoracic Injuries

Thoracic injuries account for 75% of all trauma-related deaths. There has been increasing prevalence of penetrating chest injuries in the US because of drug gangs and other violence. The survival rate has increased, however, because of improved prehospital and surgical care of these patients. It should be noted that any entry wound below the nipples in the front and below the inferior scapular angles in the back may in fact be abdominal injuries rather than purely chest injuries. All patients with gunshot wounds should be considered to have a retained projectile. Patients with both intrathoracic and intra-abdominal wounds have a higher chance of death from their injuries.

A penetrating chest injury can be low velocity, medium velocity, or high velocity. Low velocity injuries include knife wounds which only disrupt the areas that were penetrated. Medium and high velocity wounds will have a wider range of injury surrounding the immediate site of entry. High velocity wounds include bullet wounds and injuries from other military weapons. Blast injuries are particularly dangerous as these are the highest velocity injuries that are possible. These include injuries from grenades and landmines. They result in both mechanical and thermal injuries, making them very serious. About 40% of the trauma seen in the chest in military situations is penetrating chest trauma.

The most common injuries seen include hemothorax, hemopneumothorax, pneumothorax, and diaphragmatic rupture. Injuries that are less common include of pulmonary contusion, an open pneumothorax, and rib fractures.

For patients presenting with a tension pneumothorax, and x-ray is not indicated as a patient needs urgent treatment with a large-bore needle inserted into the space occupied by the tension pneumothorax. Sucking chest wounds need to be covered with an occlusive dressing. Hemorrhage needs to be quickly controlled and volume replenishment is indicated for cases of shock. Too much volume, however, can increase peripheral tissue edema and can increase the risk of ARDS. These complications can be minimized by using hypertonic solutions to replace fluid.

The mainstay of treatment for patients with penetrating chest trauma is a thoracotomy. The major indications for thoracotomy include a cardiac tamponade, major vascular injury, acute cardiac arrest in the emergency department, penetration of the chest wall, large air leaks from the chest wall, tracheobronchial injuries, esophageal injuries, or heart injuries. The survival rate of an emergency resuscitative thoracotomy is about 9 to 57%; however, the overall survival rate is only about 8%.

Indications for a late thoracotomy include a non-evacuated clotted hemothorax, the presence of a diaphragmatic hernia, the presence of a of aortic pseudoaneurysm, a traumatic lung abscess, tracheoesophageal fistula, or any other arteriovenous fistula.

Key Takeaways

- Chest trauma can be blunt trauma or penetrating trauma to the chest.

- The most common cause of a blunt chest trauma is a motor vehicle accident.

- The chest trauma can involve the chest wall, lungs, heart, or major vessels.

- Penetrating chest trauma usually results from a knife wound or gunshot wound; however, the most severe penetrating trauma comes from blast injuries.

Quiz

1. What is a good first test for the evaluation of chest trauma when the reach the emergency department?

    a. CT scan of the chest

    b. Ultrasound of the chest

    c. Thoracic aneurysm

    d. Magnetic resonance imaging of the chest

Answer: b. The ultrasound of the chest is a good first test to evaluate the patient with a suspected chest trauma in the emergency department. The CT scan would be the second-line test.

2. What is the most severe injury that can happen to the lung tissue?

    a. Pulmonary contusion

    b. Hemothorax

    c. Tension pneumothorax

    d. Lung laceration

Answer: c. The tension pneumothorax is considered the most severe injury to the lungs because it not only restricts oxygenation of the affected lung but it pushes on unaffected lung.

3. What is not considered a reason for urgent surgery to the chest wall or lung tissue?

    a. Empyema

    b. Uncontrolled hemothorax

    c. Disruption of chest wall integrity

    d. GI contents in chest tube

Answer: a. Empyema is considered a late reason for having surgery, while the other choices indications for urgent surgery to the chest wall or lung tissue.

4. What is the definitive treatment for flail chest in blunt chest trauma?

    a. Intubation

    b. Surgical fixation of the fragments

    c. Chest tube insertion

    d. Watchful waiting unless there is respiratory arrest

Answer: b. The treatment of choice is the surgical fixation of the fragments after intubating the patient who is likely in respiratory distress.

5. The fracture of which ribs is most associated with severe injuries to the underlying structures?

    a. First and second

    b. Fourth and fifth

    c. Seventh and eight

    d. Ninth and tenth

Answer: a. The fractures of ribs 1 and 2 involve a severe trauma with a high likelihood of underlying injuries as complications of this type of injury.

6. What is not considered a mainstay of clavicle fracture treatment?

    a. Figure-of-eight dressing

    b. Clavicle strap

    c. Surgical plates

    d. Sling to the ipsilateral arm

Answer: c. Surgery is rarely required for clavicle fractures and is reserved for severely displace fractures.

7. At which intercostal space should a large-bore needle be inserted in cases of tension pneumothorax?

    a. First

b. Second

c. Fourth

d. Seventh

Answer: b. A large-bore needle should be inserted in the second intercostal space at the midclavicular line in order to relieve the tension seen in tension pneumothoraces.

8. Why would a clotted hemothorax require surgery?

a. Only if the patient has ongoing dyspnea

b. To prevent further bleeding from occurring

c. To prevent fibrothorax from developing

d. To prevent a late-onset pneumothorax

Answer: c. The main reasons to do surgery on a clotted hemothorax include the prevention of empyema and fibrothorax.

9. What is the main finding in a tracheal disruption that clinches the diagnosis of the condition?

a. Subcutaneous air anteriorly

b. Shortness of breath

c. Inspiratory and expiratory stridor

d. Dysphonia

Answer: a. A finding of subcutaneous air is pathognomonic of a tracheal disruption in blunt traumatic injuries to the chest.

10. What is the best way to provide volume resuscitation in a chest trauma patient at risk for ARDS?

a. Give blood products rather than IV colloidal products

b. Use hypertonic solutions to replace lost volume

c. Do not give IV fluids to these types of patents

d. Use vasopressors instead of IV fluids

Answer: b. The best way to replace volume in a patient at risk for ARDS is to use a hypertonic solution, which causes less tissue edema.

Chapter 9: Abdominal Trauma

Because there are many vital organs in the abdomen and pelvis, trauma to these areas is hardly ever benign. The patient with abdominal trauma can have damage to any of the solid organs in the abdomen or any part of the abdominal viscus. Infections tend to be common late manifestations of abdominal trauma as the viscus of the abdomen carries billions of microorganisms—some of them pathogenic. The purpose of this chapter is to discuss the basics of abdominal trauma and its management.

Blunt Abdominal Trauma

Blunt abdominal trauma is a major cause of morbidity and fatalities among people of all ages. The abdomen is a large cavity so the problem of identifying one or more specific pathological injuries can be daunting, especially when the patient is unconscious or cannot specifically localize a site of abdominal pain. Some abdominal pathologies are relatively asymptomatic in the beginning so the exact pathology might not be picked up on the initial assessment but will declare itself over time.

The phenomenon of blunt abdominal trauma occurs during a direct collision between the injured individual and something in the environment or to acceleration-deceleration forces, which act on fixed abdominal structures. There are three major mechanisms of injury: 1) Rapid deceleration that creates a shear force within the abdomen. This causes disruption of solid and hollow organs within the abdomen (especially at fixed points along the organ's structure), 2) crush forces, where the intra-abdominal contents are crushed between the vertebral column or thoracic rib cage and the anterior abdominal wall (this causes the greatest damage to the liver, spleen, and kidneys), and 3) external compression by a lap belt or anything else that increases the intra-abdominal pressure, rupturing hollow organs.

The most frequently injured organs are the liver and the spleen, followed by injuries to the small and large intestines. CT scanning has revealed that the liver is the most commonly-injured organ, although it doesn't always rise to the level of needing any acute treatment. The rise in these injures is attributable to increased detection of minor injuries by CT scanning techniques.

The vast majority of blunt abdominal injuries stem from a motor vehicle accident. These account for up to 75 percent of all cases of abdominal trauma. Other causes include falls, industrial accidents, and sports-related accidents. Rare causes include trauma secondary to CPR or the Heimlich maneuver.

The physical examination of the injured patient is unreliable as the patient may be obtunded or intoxicated at the time of the examination. Furthermore, the patient may have other pain that takes over the patient's attention, diverting it away from abdominal pain, which may be life-threatening but not very severe in initial presentation.

The clinical assessment of the patient with abdominal pain can be difficult and can yield inaccurate results. The typical symptoms suggesting a blunt abdominal trauma include abdominal pain, tenderness of the abdomen to palpation, blood in the stool, hypovolemic shock, and peritoneal signs (like rebound tenderness and rigidity of the abdomen).

Unfortunately, it takes a large accumulation of blood in the peritoneal cavity before significant abdominal findings will be elicited. Some signs that may point to blood in the peritoneal cavity from blunt abdominal trauma include bradycardia, seat belt marks on the abdomen (seen in rupture of the small intestine), contusions shaped like a steering wheel, bruising in the umbilical area (called a Cullen sign), bruising of the flank (called the Grey Turner sign), distention of the abdomen, and the finding of bowel sounds on chest auscultation (from an abdominal diaphragmatic hernia or rupture). Crepitation or deformity of the lower rib cage suggests the possibility of a splenic or hepatic injury.

The first thing to consider in evaluating the patient with possible abdominal trauma is whether or not the patient is hemodynamically stable. If there is evidence of hemodynamic instability, urgent testing for the presence of a hemoperitoneum should be done. This involves a diagnostic peritoneal lavage (DPL) or a FAST (Focused Assessment with Sonography for Trauma) evaluation, both of which are fairly sensitive in picking up bleeding in the peritoneal cavity. Things like the CT scan or MRI scan of the abdomen should be reserved for patients who are hemodynamically stable. A flat and upright abdominal X-ray can look for free air but should be reserved for hemodynamically-stable patients.

The diagnostic peritoneal lavage or DPL is a good test for patients with unexplained shock that might be from intraabdominal bleeding and in patients who don't have the mentation to tell the providers that they have abdominal tenderness. This includes head-injured patients and intoxicated patients. Patients who require emergency surgery for other reasons should have a DPL examination to make sure they aren't bleeding in their belly as a secondary injury to the one being treated surgically.

The FAST examination can be done on just about any trauma patient, looking for hemoperitoneum. There are four windows that are assessed (the peri-cardiac window, the peri-hepatic window, the peri-splenic window, and the pelvic window). If free fluid is found anywhere in these windows, the test is positive and further investigation is warranted.

The CT scan is the gold standard test for the detection of solid organ injuries of the abdomen. It provides for sensitive and specific images of the duodenum, pancreas, liver, spleen, and genitourinary tract. It can detect the source of the bleeding in most cases, which is not the case in the DPL or FAST evaluations.

Management of Blunt Abdominal Trauma

The management of blunt abdominal trauma can be conservative (non-operative) or surgical. The patient is managed from the time they are seen by EMS personnel through to their definitive treatment at the receiving hospital or tertiary care center. After the diagnosis of blunt abdominal trauma and the finding of the source of the trauma, the surgeon may elect to do a laparotomy. The laparotomy is sometimes the definitive treatment for the trauma.

The main indications for doing a laparotomy in blunt abdominal trauma include having classic findings of peritonitis, hypovolemic shock believed to be secondary to abdominal hemorrhaging, hemodynamic instability with deterioration of the vital signs and clinical picture, and positive evidence of hemoperitoneum on FAST examination or on DPL evaluation (even though the source might not be known).

The current standard of care is to try and treat as many patients with abdominal trauma using nonoperative care. Many pediatric patients can be treated nonoperatively by transfusing blood products to keep up with intra-abdominal blood loss until the bleeding spontaneously stops. Any patient with a solid organ injury who is hemodynamically stable in be treated nonoperatively. Rarely, a splenic artery embolization can be performed in adults with splenic injury. These patients need continuous monitoring of their vital signs to make sure they remain hemodynamically stable.

It should be noted that not every patient with a positive FAST scan needs to have an emergency laparotomy. Patients who are hemodynamic stable can have a CT scan of the abdomen, which will determine the location and extent of their bleeding. It is inappropriate to do a laparotomy on every positive patient as many really do not require surgery.

Prior to arriving at the emergency department, the initial (primary) survey and secondary survey should be able to identify those patients who have life-threatening intra-abdominal injuries. These patients need urgent transport to a trauma facility that has the capability to do operative management on the traumatized patient. The airway needs to be secured and a large-bore IV needs to be placed with volume resuscitation to include colloid solution. Lactated Ringer's solution or normal saline are appropriate first line resuscitative agents. Fluids should be given as soon as the IV is started.

It is important to triage these patients carefully. The odds of death are nearly 4 times greater for critically ill patients who are sent to a nontrauma center versus a trauma center for severe traumatic injuries to the abdomen. This means that taking the patient to the closest facility may not be appropriate if this is not a trauma facility.

It is important to make sure these patients have adequate oxygenation on the way to the hospital. This may mean intubating the patient and it means maintaining an oxygen saturation level greater than 92%. Any external bleeding should be managed with direct pressure. Any time there is evidence of hemorrhagic shock without an obvious source, intra-abdominal bleeding should be considered the most likely cause of the shock. In giving IV fluids to these patients, the IV rate should be titrated to the blood pressure with the goal of a systolic blood pressure being approximately 90 mmHg, which is the amount necessary to perfused the end organs. A mast trouser should only be used in rural settings when a pelvic fracture is suspected.

In the emergency department, things like airway and breathing take precedence over abdominal trauma. Once these are managed, the abdominal injury can be assessed and managed. All of this needs to take place with adequate cervical spine protection until the cervical spine is cleared by CT scan or lateral neck x-ray.

In addressing hemorrhage in the emergency department, blood should be drawn for typing and crossmatch and O-negative blood should be available. There is only so much that crystalloid solution can do. Second large-bore IV should be placed with central lines reserved for patients who have poor peripheral venous access. If crystalloid solution has been given without success, O-negative blood should be given unless typed and crossmatched blood is available. This should be given after 2 L of fluid have been given to the patient without resolution of their hemodynamic instability.

In actuality, the first imaging studies that should be given in suspected blunt abdominal trauma patients is the chest x-ray, AP pelvic x-ray, and lateral cervical spine x-ray. This is shortly followed by a FAST examination of the chest and abdomen. If this ultrasound evaluation is equivocal or negative and the patient is still hemodynamically unstable, a DPL should be performed. If this is equivocal, serial exams can be obtained or the patient can have a CT scan of the abdomen.

Even severe solid organ injuries can be treated nonoperatively if the patient is hemodynamically stable. The same is not true of traumatic diaphragmatic injuries and ruptures of hallow organs, which generally always need laparotomy. Angiography is a good modality to use in nonoperative management of intra-abdominal injuries. Some patients can have minimally invasive arterial embolization performed in order to stop the bleeding artery. This is often done for splenic injuries.

A rarely used operative technique is called the resuscitative thoracotomy. It is used for patients with intra-abdominal trauma who are imminently dying. It is used more often for penetrating trauma than for blunt trauma. It involves opening the chest cavity and clamping the aorta in order to provide lifesaving blood flow to the brain and heart. It gives the surgeon the opportunity to repair any intra-abdominal injury before restoring blood flow to the abdomen. It is rarely of any benefit to the patient who has already suffered a cardiac arrest or who has no signs of life. The lesser goals of this procedure are to evacuate pericardial tamponade, to perform cardiac massage, and to control intrathoracic bleeding.

The definitive treatment for some cases of intra-abdominal blunt trauma is the laparotomy, which should be done in unstable patients, patients with peritonitis, patients who are deteriorating, and in patients with hemoperitoneum. Broad-spectrum antibiotics should be given to avoid sepsis. The first part of this procedure involves packing all four quadrants of the abdomen, removing existing clots, and clamping bleeding blood vessels. This is followed by a meticulous examination of the abdomen and repair of any structures that can be repaired. The retroperitoneum and pelvis should be inspected at this time. Small stable hematomas around the kidneys should be left intact as should any pelvic hematomas. External fixation should be used for pelvic fractures.

While there is extra cost in doing an exploratory laparotomy, a negative laparotomy has not been found to increase mortality. For this reason, it is better to do an exploratory laparotomy and have it be negative than to avoid this procedure and a possibly hemorrhaging patient. Even so, the CT scan of the abdomen has largely replaced the diagnostic laparotomy in the evaluation of equivocal patients.

Prognosis for patients with blunt abdominal trauma is very good. Excluding patients who die at the scene, only about 5 to 10% of patients will die after reaching the hospital. Of these, only about a fourth of patients actually have the cause of death being their abdominal traumatic injuries.

Key Takeaways

- Blunt abdominal trauma carries significant morbidity and mortality in adults and pediatric patients.

- Most blunt abdominal traumatic injuries are secondary to motor vehicle accidents.

- The most sensitive ways of determining intra-abdominal bleeding include DPL and the FAST examination.

- The current standard of care is nonoperative management of intra-abdominal injuries unless there is an obvious reason to do a laparotomy.

Quiz

1. What finding is least likely to identify a patient as having abdominal pathology in a situation of possible blunt abdominal trauma?

   a. Abdominal pain

   b. Rigidity of the abdomen

   c. Nausea and vomiting

   d. Tenderness to palpation

Answer: c. All of the above are signs that there might be internal injuries from blunt abdominal trauma except for nausea and vomiting, which is nonspecific and can occur in the absence of abdominal trauma.

2. You identify a patient as having a positive Cullen sign. What does this mean?

    a. Bruising around the umbilicus

    b. Right upper quadrant abdominal rigidity

    c. Rebound tenderness in all four quadrants

    d. Flank pain on percussion of the flank

Answer: a. A positive Cullen sign is bruising around the umbilicus, which is a late sign of blood in the peritoneum.

3. What type of injury is most commonly seen when the patient has a lap belt area of ecchymosis around the lower waist?

    a. Splenic rupture

    b. Small intestinal rupture

    c. Peritonitis

    d. Hepatic rupture

Answer: b. The finding of an area of lap-belt ecchymosis most correlates with a small intestinal rupture because of its location.

4. When would a CT scan of the abdomen be preferable over a FAST examination?

    a. When the patient requires urgent abdominal surgery for probable solid organ disruption.

    b. When the source of the bleeding is needed to be determined.

    c. When the hemorrhaging is probable but the FAST exam is negative.

    d. In low risk cases, where confirmation of the lack of abdominal bleeding is necessary.

Answer: b. The CT scan is the best way of determining the actual source of any abdominal bleeding. This is the gold standard test for this purpose.

5. Which is not considered a mechanism by which trauma to the intra-abdominal structures usually occurs?

    a. Crushing injury

    b. Acceleration-deceleration

    c. Laceration by bone fragments

    d. Compression increasing abdominal pressure

Answer: c. All of the above choices lead to intra-abdominal injuries except for laceration, which would rarely be a cause of an intra-abdominal injury from blunt force trauma.

6. What is the major cause of blunt abdominal trauma in developed countries?

    a. Falls from a great height

    b. Pedestrian accidents

    c. Sports-related accidents

    d. Motor vehicle accidents

Answer: d. The most common cause of blunt abdominal trauma injuries is the motor vehicle accident. The other causes are less common than a motor vehicle accident.

7. In managing the unstable patient in the field with intra-abdominal trauma, what is a resuscitative method of choice?

    a. To give O-negative blood through a large-bore IV

    b. To apply mast trousers

    c. To give 5% dextrose solution

    d. To give a lactated Ringer's solution

Answer: d. The treatment of choice for stabilizing the patient in the field is to give lactated Ringer's solution through a large-bore IV.

8. You are caring for a patient at the scene who has been traumatized a motor vehicle accident and who has extreme hypotension without any external bleeding. What is the most likely cause of the bleeding?

    a. Thoracic trauma

    b. Pelvic bone fracture

    c. Intra-abdominal hemorrhaging

    d. Spinal shock

Answer: c. Patients with hemorrhagic shock and no obvious source should be considered to have intra-abdominal hemorrhaging until proven otherwise.

9. In titrating the blood pressure of a patient receiving IV fluids for intra-abdominal trauma, what systolic blood pressure reading should be the target reading?

    a. 120 mm Hg

    b. 110 mm Hg

    c. 100 mm Hg

    d. 90 mm Hg

Answer: d. In titrating the IV fluids, a minimum of 90 mm Hg systolic pressure should be aimed for.

10. What is performed as the major reason to do a resuscitative thoracotomy in order to save the patient's life?

    a. Cardiac massage

    b. A pericardial window

    c. Repair of any lung or heart abnormities

    d. Cross-clamping of the descending aorta

Answer: d. In a resuscitative thoracotomy, the descending aorta is cross-clamped in order to provide more oxygenated blood to the brain and heart while reparative efforts are made to correct any intra-abdominal hemorrhaging.

Chapter 10: Acute Abdomen and Pelvic Pain

This chapter is devoted to discussing the evaluation and management of the acute abdomen and the related phenomenon of pelvic pain. These are common problems in emergency medicine and require a systematic approach that attempts to distinguish between a non-operative condition and those that require surgical intervention. The definition of the "acute abdomen" is one that ultimately needs surgery to treat the patient's abdominal or pelvic complaints.

The Acute Abdomen

The evaluation of the acute abdomen can lead to the finding of a benign condition, a serious but nonoperative condition, or a surgical emergency. The evaluation starts with a history, a thorough physical examination, imaging studies, and laboratory testing. The history and physical exam may point to a likely diagnosis that will guide further evaluation modalities. For example, the finding of constipation and severe abdominal distention may indicate a bowel obstruction, while classic right lower quadrant abdominal pain often leads to a diagnosis of appendicitis.

As for imaging, the American College of Radiology has set up guidelines regarding the imaging of the abdomen. Ultrasonography is the imaging test of choice for right upper quadrant pain and pelvic pain in women of childbearing age, while CT scanning is recommended for right lower quadrant pain and left lower quadrant pain.

It should be noted abdominal pain is extremely common in the emergency department, accounting for about 5% of all emergency department visits. Of these, about 10% have a surgical abdomen or other serious abdominal problem. Because of this, a thorough evaluation of all abdominal complaints should be undertaken in the emergency department before discharging or admitting the patient.

Some important caveats to remember include the fact appendicitis is mainly a clinical evaluation so that a normal white blood cell count does not rule out the presence of the disease. In addition, all patients with epigastric pain are candidates for possible pancreatitis and should have both a serum amylase and serum lipase tested. The main imaging tests for abdominal pain are the ultrasound evaluation and the CT scan of the abdomen.

The differential diagnosis of acute abdominal pain includes a long list of problems can be benign or serious. Sometimes the location of the pain will help in the diagnosis, such as right lower quadrant abdominal pain and appendicitis. The location of the pain is the most important factor in determining how the patient is worked up. Is important to rule out serious illnesses first, such as mesenteric ischemia and dissecting aortic aneurysm, followed by surgical conditions, such as bowel rupture, cholecystitis, and appendicitis. It should be noted that some abdominal pain is from the abdominal wall itself. These conditions can be difficult to diagnose in the absence of other clinical findings.

Differential diagnosis of abdominal pain is large and includes the following:

- **Right upper quadrant abdominal pain**—biliary colic, cholelithiasis, cholecystitis, cholangitis, colitis, diverticulitis, hepatic disease (abscess, tumor, or inflammation), pulmonary embolism, pneumonia, nephrolithiasis, and pyelonephritis.

- **Epigastric abdominal pain**—cholecystitis, cholangitis, cholelithiasis, myocardial infarction, pericarditis, esophagitis, peptic ulceration, gastritis, pancreatic mass, pancreatitis, aortic dissection, mesenteric ischemia, pyelonephritis and nephrolithiasis.

- **Left upper quadrant pain**—aortic dissection, mesenteric ischemia, early appendicitis, esophagitis, peptic ulcer disease, or small bowel obstruction.

- **Left upper quadrant pain**—aortic dissection, mesenteric ischemia, diverticulitis, colitis, irritable bowel syndrome, or inflammatory bowel disease.

- **Periumbilical pain**—ectopic pregnancy, uterine fibroids, ovarian mass, pelvic inflammatory disease, nephrolithiasis, pyelonephritis, early appendicitis, esophagitis, gastritis, peptic ulcer, small-bowel mass or obstruction, aortic dissection, or mesenteric ischemia.

- **Right lower quadrant pain**—colitis, appendicitis, irritable bowel syndrome, inflammatory bowel disease, ectopic pregnancy, pelvic inflammatory disease, uterine fibroids, ovarian cancer cystitis, nephrolithiasis, or pyelonephritis.

- **Suprapubic pain**—appendicitis, colitis, diverticulitis, IBD, IBS, ectopic pregnancy, fibroids, ovarian mass, torsion, PID, cystitis, nephrolithiasis, or pyelonephritis.

- **Any location of pain**—abdominal wall causes like herpes zoster, muscle strain, or hernia. Other possibilities include bowel obstruction, mesenteric ischemia, peritonitis, narcotic withdrawal, sickle cell crisis, porphyria, IBD, or heavy metal poisoning.

The patient should never receive sedation or pain relief before obtaining a thorough history. This is because pain may be masked by either sedating the patient or giving them pain relievers. The pain should be rated on a pain scale, the location of the pain should be evaluated, the migration of the pain should be asked about, and any exacerbating or relieving factors should be noted before even touching the patient's abdomen.

Associated symptoms should be asked about. For example, the finding of obstipation highly predicts a bowel obstruction and right lower abdominal pain highly predicts appendicitis (especially if it has migrated from the periumbilical area.

Colicky abdominal pain highly points to a problem with an abdominal viscus. This type of pain comes from smooth muscle contraction secondary to a partial or complete obstruction (of the biliary tract, renal pelvis, ureters, or small bowels. The absence of colicky pain, particularly in the right upper quadrant often effectively rules out cholecystitis as the patient's final diagnosis as it is seen in more than 75 percent of cases.

The finding that the patient has an associated infection with Helicobacter pylori predicts the cause of the pain as being a duodenal or gastric ulcer. Patients who use NSAIDs on a regular basis are likely to have gastritis as a cause of their epigastric pain, even if they don't have a concurrent H. pylori infection.

The concurrent findings of these things indicate the probability of a surgical abdomen: protracted vomiting, fever, presyncope or syncope, and GI blood loss. Patients with peritonitis tend not to move very much as pain makes their symptoms worse, while patients with renal colic cannot sit still. Any fever suggests an infection but its absence doesn't rule out an infection. Orthostatic hypotension and tachycardia suggest low volume status (hypovolemia). It should be noted that upper abdominal pain may be from either the heart or lungs so these should be evaluated.

Some evaluations in the physical examination can predict the cause of the pain. The Carnett's sign involves having the supine patient lift their head and shoulders off the table, tightening the abdominal muscles and suggesting abdominal wall pain. A positive Murphy's sign will predict cholecystitis about 65 percent of the time. A positive psoas sign predicts appendicitis.

All patients with abdominal pain should have a rectal examination, Guaiac testing, and a pelvic exam unless the source of the pain is obviously the abdominal wall. Rectal examinations can show occult or gross blood in the stool, a fecal impaction, a mass in the rectal area, or retrocecal appendicitis.

A pelvic exam can evaluate the adnexa for an ectopic pregnancy or ovarian mass. The pelvic exam might show cervical motion tenderness seen in PID. Cultures of the cervix and vaginal fluids can help diagnose an infectious cause of the pain. A tubo-ovarian abscess is the likely diagnosis with fever, adnexal mass, adnexal tenderness, and a negative pregnancy test. A pregnancy test should be done on all females of reproductive age who present with abdominal pain.

The laboratory testing should be guided by the history and physical examination. Patients suspected of having an infection like appendicitis should have a CBC with differential. A high WBC count is 77 percent sensitive for appendicitis meaning that up to a fourth of patients won't have a high WBC count but will still have appendicitis. Epigastric pain mandates doing a serum lipase and amylase test. Liver chemistries are necessary for right upper quadrant abdominal pain. Urinalysis should be done on patients with flank pain, dysuria, or hematuria. Women at risk for STDs should have a chlamydia and gonorrhea test in evaluating them for PID.

The imaging studies for the evaluation of the acute abdomen depend on the location of the pain. Ultrasounds, radionuclide testing, CT testing, and even a flat plate and upright evaluations are possible choices for imaging in cases of acute abdominal pain.

The following are the recommended imaging tests of choice for patients with differing locations of abdominal pain:

- **Right upper quadrant pain**—ultrasound

- **Left upper quadrant pain**—CT scan without contrast or upper GI series

- **Right lower quadrant pain**—CT scan with contrast

- **Left lower contrast**—CT with oral and IV contrast

- **Suprapubic**—ultrasound

A plain x-ray, such as a flat and upright evaluation of the abdomen can be helpful when looking for free air under the diaphragm, such as would be seen with a rupture of a viscus. Calcified stones, such as gallstones or kidney stones, can be seen on an x-ray image. About 10% of gallstones, 5% of appendicoliths, and 90% of kidney stones will contain calcium. In addition, a bowel obstruction with dilated loops of ileus and air-fluid levels can be seen in paralytic ileus.

In a pregnant woman with abdominal pain, exposure to radiation should be avoided. For this reason, an ultrasound is recommended for any lower abdominal or pelvic pain in pregnancy. If an ectopic pregnancy is suspected, the ultrasound should be a transvaginal ultrasound as this is highly sensitive and specific for the detection of this pregnancy complication. In fact, the sensitivity of detecting an ectopic pregnancy in a woman who has laboratory confirmation of a pregnancy is 95 percent.

Acute Abdomen in Pregnancy

Pregnant women can have abdominal pain that is pregnancy-related, gynecologically-related, or non-gynecologically-related. For this reason, there is an overlap of specialties necessary for caring for these women. The cause for an acute abdomen can be anything that happens to coincide with being pregnant and may or may not actually be associated with the pregnancy. The diagnostic choices are often very similar to that seen in non-pregnant patients except that there are a few pregnancy-related choices to consider. The workup is complicated by the fact that x-ray imaging should be avoided if possible in a pregnant woman, making the diagnosis harder to identify. Pregnant women naturally have elevated WBC counts, which make this a difficult test to interpret.

Women can have just about any incidental cause of an acute abdomen or acute abdominal pain that is unrelated to the pregnancy, including an acute appendicitis, peptic ulcer disease, acute pancreatitis, gastroenteritis, hepatitis, pancreatic pseudocyst, diverticulitis, toxic megacolon, hernia, bowel perforation, or bowel obstruction.

Genitourinary causes of acute abdominal pain in a pregnant woman might be secondary to a ruptured ovarian cyst, torsion of the ovary/adnexa, renal or ureteral stone, ruptured renal pelvis, or ureteral obstruction.

Vascular causes of an acute abdomen in a pregnant woman can include mesenteric venous thrombosis, superior mesenteric artery syndrome, ruptured aneurysm, or splenic artery aneurysm. A pulmonary embolism can result in abdominal pain, which is more common in pregnancy.

Pregnancy-related causes of acute abdominal pain include acute cholecystitis, acute cystitis, acute cystitis, pyelonephritis, fatty liver of pregnancy, ruptured rectus abdominis muscle, or uterine torsion. Early in the pregnancy, abdominal pain can be secondary to a ruptured ectopic pregnancy, septic abortion (with secondary peritonitis), retroverted uterus causing urinary tract obstruction. Later in pregnancy, there can be torsion or degeneration of myomata, placental abruption, placenta accreta, uterine rupture, chorioamnionitis, or HELLP syndrome (hemolysis, elevated liver function tests, and low platelets).

In diagnostic imaging of acute abdominal pain in pregnancy, ultrasound should be the imaging test of choice, regardless of the location of the pain. If a CT scan is necessary, it should be done without hesitation as there is no evidence that a single dose of radiation such as would be received in a CT scan is harmful to the fetus. MRI scanning is not at all harmful in pregnancy and can be used as a good substitute for any test for which a CT scan would be otherwise indicated.

In treating the acute abdomen during pregnancy, the indications for emergency surgery do not change just because the patient is pregnant. Second-trimester surgery is safest of all the times for having a semi-elective surgery as the risk to the fetus is lower and the risk for things like preterm delivery is also low. Laparoscopy can be very successful as a minimally-invasive way to manage simple things like appendicitis in pregnancy. There is a shorter hospital stay, easier ambulation after surgery, earlier ability to tolerate oral intake, and a decreased need for narcotic analgesia with laparoscopic surgery.

The biggest risk for any pregnant woman with an acute abdomen is preterm labor and delivery. Treating these patients prophylactically with tocolytic medications has not been found to be helpful.

Glucocorticoid therapy should be considered if preterm delivery is likely to occur; however, they should be used with caution if there is the possibility of a major infection.

The most common non-obstetric cause of an acute abdomen in pregnancy is appendicitis. Pregnancy does not increase the rate of appendicitis but does increase the risk of complications, with a 25 percent risk of perforation. For this reason, surgery to remove the appendix should occur as soon as it is identified as any delays in surgery will increase the risk of perforation.

Another common non-obstetric cause of a surgical abdomen in pregnancy is acute cholecystitis. Asymptomatic disease is extremely common in pregnancy but actual inflammation and perforation of the gallbladder are much rarer conditions. These women often present with recurrent episodes of biliary colic and will have vomiting when the gallbladder becomes inflamed. Tenderness is usually found in the right upper quadrant. The patient can be treated with supportive therapy, including NG suction and antibiotics; however, if this fails, a semi-emergency surgery is indicated. Laparoscopic cholecystectomy procedures are safe in pregnancy.

Acute pancreatitis is fortunately very rare in pregnancy and is usually secondary to cholelithiasis. Less common causes include alcohol abuse, elevated triglycerides, abdominal trauma, viral infections, and hyperparathyroidism. These patients present with epigastric pain, severe nausea and vomiting, and diminished bowel sounds. The serum amylase is the best diagnostic lab test for this disorder as it is elevated when the pancreas is inflamed. The treatment is mainly supportive and not surgical. The glucose and electrolyte levels should be monitored and corrected. The patient must be NPO with continuous gastric suctioning. Total parenteral nutrition should be considered in protracted cases.

Intestinal obstruction is also an uncommon occurrence. It occurs mainly in the second or third trimester and is usually secondary to prior abdominal surgery and intra-abdominal adhesions. Less likely, a volvulus can be the cause of the blockage. Very rare causes of intestinal obstruction in pregnancy include intussusception, incarcerated inguinal hernia, or incarcerated femoral hernia. Vomiting occurs in proximal obstructions, while pain is the main feature in distal obstructions. A flat plate and X-ray the abdomen can be done in pregnancy with relative safety and will show the area of obstruction. The most effective treatment for this is surgery, even in the gravid patient. The mortality rate is as high as 20 percent.

Kidney stones and ureteral stones can cause abdominal pain in pregnancy. The two most common complaints include flank pain and vomiting. Gross hematuria will likely be present with a fourth of all patients having a prior history of stones. A coexisting UTI may be present. The workup includes a urinalysis and an ultrasound of the ureters to rule out an obstruction. Most stones will pass spontaneously with hydration as the only treatment.

Gynecological and obstetric causes of abdominal pain in pregnancy include ruptured ovarian cysts, adnexal torsion, degeneration of myomata (occurring mainly in the second trimester), placental abruption (occurring in one out of 150 deliveries), uterine rupture (occurring in one out of 3000 pregnancies), and hepatic rupture (extremely rare and associated with HELLP syndrome).

Key Takeaways

- The acute abdomen is, by definition, abdominal pain and other symptoms that are secondary to a problem that generally requires surgical correction.

- The diagnosis of abdominal pain requires a thorough history, physical examination, lab work, and imaging.

- The differential diagnosis of acute abdominal pain is large and encompasses several organ systems.

- The imaging test of choice is dependent upon the location of the abdominal pain.

- The pregnant patient may have abdominal pain related to the pregnancy, related to a non-pregnancy gynecological condition, or related to something other than pregnancy.

Quiz

1. What is the diagnostic test of choice for right upper quadrant abdominal pain?

   a. FAST evaluation

   b. Ultrasound of the right upper quadrant

   c. CT scan of the chest and abdomen

   d. Flat and upright X-ray abdomen

Answer: b. The diagnostic test of choice for right upper quadrant abdominal pain is the ultrasound of the affected area.

2. What is the diagnostic imaging test of choice for the patient with left lower quadrant abdominal pain?

   a. FAST evaluation

   b. Ultrasound of the right upper quadrant

   c. CT scan of the abdomen

   d. Flat and upright X-ray the abdomen

Answer: c. The diagnostic imaging test of choice in left or right lower quadrant abdominal pain is a CT scan of the abdomen.

3. What percentage of patients with abdominal pain in the emergency department will have a serious surgical abdomen?

   a. 1 percent

   b. 10 percent

   c. 25 percent

d. 40 percent

Answer: b. About 10% of patients presenting to the emergency department with abdominal pain will have a serious surgical abdomen or other life-threatening cause of abdominal pain.

4. What associated finding has the highest predictive value in determining that the patient's pain is from a bowel obstruction?

   a. Blood in the stool

   b. Fever

   c. Obstipation

   d. Nausea and vomiting

Answer: c. Obstipation has the highest predictive value in determining that the patient's pain is secondary to a bowel obstruction.

5. Which abdominal area is least likely to yield colicky abdominal pain?

   a. Biliary tract

   b. Ureters

   c. Small intestines

   d. Esophagus

Answer: d. Any of the above may be partially or totally obstructed, leading to colicky pain except for the esophagus, which doesn't yield this classic type of abdominal pain.

6. An infection with which pathogen is linked to the development of duodenal ulcers?

   a. Rotavirus

   b. Helicobacter pylori

   c. Listeria species

   d. Salmonella species

Answer: b. Patients with abdominal pain who have known Helicobacter pylori infections are at a higher risk of their pain being secondary to a duodenal or gastric ulcer.

7. What testing should be done on all women between the ages of about 13 and 50 who present with abdominal pain?

   a. Serum antibodies for gonorrhea and chlamydia

   b. Vaginal swab for Candida species

   c. Serum HCG test

   d. Pelvic ultrasound

Answer: c. A serum HCG test should be done on all women of childbearing age who present with abdominal pain as pregnancy can change the differential diagnosis greatly.

8. What testing should be done on female patients with lower abdominal pain, fever, and cervical motion tenderness?

    a. Chlamydia

    b. Gardnerella vaginalis

    c. Candida

    d. Syphilis

Answer: a. Both chlamydia and gonorrhea testing should be done on suspected PID cases as these are the two main causes of this problem.

9. The patient you are evaluating is experiencing left upper quadrant abdominal pain. What imaging test would be the imaging test of choice for this?

    a. Ultrasonography

    b. Upper GI series

    c. MRI of the abdomen

    d. CT scan with contrast

Answer: b. The patient's choices for left upper quadrant abdominal pain imaging include a CT scan without contrast ro an upper GI series.

10. What is the most common cause of an acute surgical abdomen in a pregnant woman that is not related to pregnancy?

    a. Acute appendicitis

    b. Acute cholecystitis

    c. Acute pancreatitis

    d. Perforated gastric ulcer

Answer: a. Acute appendicitis occurs at the same rate whether the patient is pregnant or not; however, the complication rate in pregnancy is higher when compared to the non-pregnant patient.

Chapter 11: Multiple Trauma Care

It is not uncommon for the emergency room physician to encounter a patient who has the confounding problem of having multiple areas of trauma secondary to a motor vehicle accident, a fall, or other serious injury. These patients need to be managed in a manner that addresses the more serious problems first, followed by a systematic assessment and management of the less serious injuries. The care of the multiply-injured patient is the focus of this chapter.

Overview

The evaluation of the critically-injured trauma patient with multiple areas of bodily trauma can be challenging. Patients can die from any number of traumatic injuries and it is often difficult to determine which traumatic injury to attend to first. Mortality can happen immediately (at the scene), early in the course of treatment (in the emergency department or soon after admission), or late after the trauma (days or weeks after the injury).

Most immediate deaths cannot be prevented and occur before the patient is evaluated. Early deaths occur within a few minutes to hours after the accident, with the main cause being hemorrhage and secondary cardiovascular collapse. Late trauma deaths happen days to weeks after the trauma with the major cause of death being sepsis and secondary multiple organ failure. Rural patients tend to have a higher rate of early deaths when compared to urban patients.

Early deaths can also happen secondary to massive CNS injuries or to lack of oxygenation of vital organs. Impaired ventilation can result in lack of tissue oxygenation and circulatory collapse from hemorrhaging can result in a lack of end-organ perfusion. Anything that disrupts the drive to breathe (such as a brainstem injury) will impair ventilation.

According to Advanced Trauma Life Support protocol, the first step in the management of the multiply-injured patient is to quickly identify those injuries that are life-threatening. Next comes the initiation of support of the vital cardiorespiratory systems. Finally, there is the identification and performance of definitive therapy or transfer to a trauma facility that can provide definitive care.

Triage involves the prioritization of patients, treating those patients with the highest likelihood of deterioration first. It takes into consideration the patient's vital signs, mechanism of injury, and underlying medical conditions. Extremes of age, multiple injuries, neurological injuries, and having preexisting illnesses put a patient higher on the triage list. Patients not expected to survive regardless of intervention are not placed high on the triage list.

The triage process when resources are limited is more difficult. It takes into account the number of qualified providers available to handle the totality of traumatic injuries. In some cases, the goal of triage is to maximize the number of surviving patients given the available resources. It may mean choosing not to prioritize a more critically-injured patient because there are no resources available to handle such a traumatic injury.

The treating trauma team should be led by a provider with the most experience handling trauma cases, with midlevel practitioners and less skilled physicians resourced to handle the patient airways, perform IV insertions, obtain blood samples, monitor vital signs, and perform the secondary surveys. Consultants in neurology, orthopedics, and general surgery should be notified and, if possible, enlisted to care for the trauma patient as soon as possible. Neurosurgery is particularly warranted as early neurosurgical care can dramatically affect the patient's survival rate with the least amount of disability.

More people die from rural injuries than die from urban injuries, even with adequately-trained ATLS personnel caring for the patient. These patients have a delay in getting to any hospital and an even greater delay in getting to a facility that provides tertiary trauma care. Injuries tend to be more severe in rural areas and there is an extreme lack of trauma centers in rural areas. The answer to the problem doesn't include increasing the number of rural trauma centers as the numbers of patients seen in trauma centers need to be high in order to have a better survival rate.

Care of the Trauma Patient

The initial care of the trauma patient starts with the primary survey, which is the assessment of the most life-threatening injuries. This should be done as quickly as possible and should be followed by resuscitation of the patient's cardiorespiratory system. Absolute diagnostic certainty is not required until after the patient has been resuscitated. If there is a lack of available rescuers, nothing in the secondary survey should be addressed until the patient has been adequately resuscitated and life-threatening injuries have been treated.

The major steps of the primary survey include the ABCDE steps, which starts with airway and then proceeds sequentially with breathing, circulation, disability (neurological outcome), and exposure/environment. The airway is assessed by determining the patency of the patient's air passages. The airway may be obstructed secondary to direct trauma, lack of consciousness of the patient, bleeding in the airway, or foreign bodies in the airway. Simple suctioning, the jaw-thrust maneuver, or endotracheal intubation can address the airway. Facial trauma may necessitate the placement of a surgical airway.

The evaluation of breathing involves seeing if the patient is oxygenated and ventilating properly. The absence of spontaneous breathing is determined after the airway is made patent. A pneumothorax or malposition of the endotracheal tube can impair ventilation. A tension pneumothorax should be identified and treated as soon as possible. Mobility of the chest wall from trauma can impair the patient's oxygenation and ventilatory capacity. The treatment of choice for ventilation impairment is mechanical ventilation using positive-pressure ventilation. This is true regardless of the cause of the ventilatory failure.

Circulation in the trauma patient involves evaluating vital signs, looking for evidence of hypovolemia, looking for external bleeding sources, evaluating the patient or cardiac tamponade, and looking at the extremities to see if the patient is perfusing their periphery. The treatment of choice for hemorrhaging is to place two large-bore IVs and run in lactated Ringer solution to keep the blood pressure at a level that is perfusing the vital organs. This is usually a systolic BP of at least 90 mm Hg. Pericardiocentesis is the treatment of choice for cardiac tamponade. Direct pressure should be applied to any external bleeding sources.

The patient's level of disability is determined by assessing the patient's mental status and their degree of motor abilities. A brief assessment using the Glasgow Coma Scale score is the best way to evaluate the patient's neurological impairment. The pupils should be examined for symmetry in movement when a light is shined into the eyes. Spinal cord trauma can be assessed by a brief peripheral motor examination.

Impending herniation of the brainstem can be assumed if there is significant difference in pupil size, a lack of pupillary light reflexes, or obvious hemiplegia. Any of these findings indicate the urgent need for hyperventilation, hypertonic saline, IV mannitol, and immediate neurosurgical consult.

If there is any possibility of a spinal cord injury, the entire spinal column needs to be immobilized. While most traumatic injuries occur in the cervical spine, a lower spinal injury can still occur and can still lead to paraplegia or other distal neurological deficit. Endotracheal intubation is indicated for any high spinal cord injuries.

The last step in the primary survey involves patient exposure and the control of the victim's immediate environment. The entirety of the patient's clothing should be removed for a thorough head-to-toe evaluation. At the same time, the patient should be prevented from becoming hypothermic in the process. This involves using warmed intravenous fluids, heat lamps, and warming blankets. The possibility of hypothermia can exist even after the patient is moved indoors.

As the primary survey is being done, ECG leads should be placed, a pulse oximeter should be applied, and a blood pressure cuff should be applied. The stomach should be decompressed to decrease the aspiration risk. A urinary catheter should be inserted to monitor the fluid resuscitation efforts as urine output is the best way to assess the patient's response to these efforts.

Resuscitation starts as soon as a compromise in the patient's status is recognized and continues until the patient is stable enough to have a secondary survey performed. The vital signs are continuously monitored, and the airway is continually addressed and managed. In doing volume resuscitation, several liters of crystalloid may need to be given in the first 24 hours after the injury. Blood should be given if there is inadequate response to crystalloid solution. Surgery may be necessary if resuscitation efforts fail to maintain the patient's vital signs. The end of resuscitation is marked by continuously normal vital signs, a lack of obvious blood loss, an acceptable urine output, and normal end-organ function. ABGs may be necessary to assess the patient's oxygenation.

The secondary survey involves a head-to-toe evaluation that is begun only after resuscitative efforts are complete. This involves an identification of all of the patient's obvious injuries. The primary survey is repeated first to make sure the patient has responded to the resuscitation phase. This also identifies any deterioration that may have taken place.

The patient's history should be taken from the patient or from bystanders. Preexisting medical issues, medications taken, allergies, time of last meal, tetanus status, and trauma-related events should be evaluated. A head-to-toe evaluation of the patient's status should be undertaken, looking for obvious and occult injuries. The patient's back should be evaluated by log-rolling the patient to look for injuries not obvious in the supine patient. A detailed cranial nerve evaluation should take place as part of a complete neurological evaluation.

The chest, abdomen, and pelvis should be evaluated visually and using palpation to look for distension, edema, crepitation, or deformities. If there is penetrating trauma, entry and exit points should be looked for and documented. The extremities should be visualized and palpated for obvious long bone fractures that might need stabilization. X-rays, if available, should be done on the chest, the lateral cervical spine, and of any areas of extremity abnormalities. The patient's peripheral and central nervous system should be continuously evaluated. The most common and most important imaging study needed on the trauma patient is the AP chest x-ray.

Other important imaging studies that need to be done on trauma patients include the AP pelvis film (which can show areas that may be occultly hemorrhaging), the cervical spine series (especially the lateral cervical spine x-ray), and the FAST examination (which is an ultrasound assessment of the pericardium, the abdomen, the chest, and the pelvis).

Doing an extensive imaging routine on a patient who doesn't have the availability of a surgeon or other specialist to act on the results is not cost-effective and only delays the time it takes for the patient to be transported to a definitive care destination. These studies should be deferred until the patient reaches the tertiary care center.

The definitive radiologic study for trauma patients is the CT scan. It can be performed on the head, cervical spine, chest, pelvis, and abdomen and is the best non-invasive tool for identifying major areas of injury without having to do a surgical exploration. CT scanning should be done when the patient is stable and should be done on all areas where trauma is suspected. It is not very helpful, however, for extremity injuries and plain radiography is usually all that is necessary in these situations. CT scanning has largely replaced plain radiography for spinal injuries at all levels.

Angiography can be done for diagnostic and therapeutic reasons in the trauma patient. It can be helpful in identifying the sites of major arterial bleeding, especially in areas that are not otherwise accessible. For retroperitoneal injuries and pelvic bleeding, the angiogram can be used to embolize major vessels that are bleeding, with control of the bleeding faster than can be done surgically. Angiography and embolization can also be done on liver injuries, spleen injuries, and kidney injuries.

The most important blood test obtained in a trauma situation is the type and crossmatch, which may be necessary acutely in order to have type-specific and matched blood available for the hemorrhaging patient. Arterial blood gases might be helpful initially but pulse oximetry has taken the place of routinely doing this blood test. A baseline hematocrit is useful on admission but it may be normal, even in the face of severe hemorrhaging. It isn't until fluid resuscitation occurs that the hematocrit will begin to all. Urine toxicology screens and blood alcohol screens are helpful if the trauma patient has a decreased level of consciousness.

Key Takeaways

- The first part of assessing the trauma patient is the primary survey, which looks exclusively for life-threatening injuries.

- The biggest thing impacting a patient's survival from a traumatic injury is the time to arrival at a trauma center for definitive care.

- The assessment of the trauma patient follows the ABCDEs of assessment, which starts with the airway and proceeds to breathing, circulation, disability, and exposure/environment.

- The definitive radiologic study in the evaluation of the trauma patient is the CT scan, which can be done on most traumatized body areas.

Quiz

1. What is considered the main cause of death among patients who die early after a traumatic injury?

    a. Neurological injury

    b. Respiratory failure

    c. Hemorrhaging

    d. Respiratory compromise

Answer: c. The most common cause of death in early post-traumatic cases is hemorrhaging that causes secondary cardiovascular collapse.

2. What is the most common cause of late-trauma deaths in a multiply-injured patient?

    a. Postoperative complications

    b. Sepsis

    c. Neurological injury

    d. ARDS

Answer: b. Sepsis and secondary multiple organ failure is the most common cause of death in patients who die late in the course of their recovery from a multiple trauma.

3. Which patient is least likely to be placed high on the list when triaging a multiple-patient accident?

    a. An infant with respiratory distress

    b. An elderly patient with chest trauma and a history of COPD

    c. A middle-aged patient with a cervical spine injury

    d. A young person with massive chest trauma and no vital signs

Answer: d. The patient with massive chest trauma and no vital signs has virtually no chance of survival so they are least likely to be addressed if there are other patients that have a better chance of survival but are also critically injured.

4. What aspect of the primary survey is addressed first when assessing the multiple trauma patient?

    a. Airway

    b. Breathing

    c. Hemorrhaging

    d. Neurological impairment

Answer: a. The airway takes precedence over all of the other assessments in the primary survey and should always be addressed first.

5. What is the main reason why a patient would need a surgical airway in a multiple-trauma situation?

   a. Lack of respiratory drive to breathe secondary to CNS impairment.

   b. Cervical spine injury

   c. Severe maxillofacial trauma

   d. Bleeding in the nose or mouth

Answer: c. The most obvious reason to place a surgical airway is when the patient has severe maxillofacial trauma that impairs the ability to see or gain access to the vocal cords or the oropharynx.

6. What is the treatment of choice in patients who are not adequately ventilating despite a patent airway?

   a. Evaluate and treat any tension pneumothoraces.

   b. Positive-pressure ventilation

   c. Reposition the patient to maximize airway patency

   d. Intubation of the patient

Answer: b. Regardless of the cause of the ventilatory failure, the treatment of choice is positive-pressure ventilation, which may or may not necessitate intubation.

7. What is the most accurate way of assessing the trauma patient's response to volume expansion?

   a. Assessing the pulse rate

   b. Monitoring the amount of colloidal fluids given over time

   c. Following the urine output

   d. Continuous pulse oximetry reading monitoring

Answer: c. The urine output is the best way to assess the trauma patient's response to volume expansion in the resuscitation efforts.

8. What is not considered an end-point in the patient's resuscitation after multiple trauma?

   a. A lack of obvious bleeding

   b. An adequate urine output

   c. Normal vital signs

   d. Return to normal consciousness

Answer: d. The patient does not have to return to normal consciousness to be considered having reached the endpoint of resuscitation. The other parameters are factors in the endpoint of resuscitation.

9. What is the most important imaging study to be obtained on a trauma patient?

    a. CT of the head

    b. Cervical spine studies

    c. AP chest x-ray

    d. Pelvic bone x-ray

Answer: c. The most important imaging study to obtain on a patient who is traumatically-injured is the AP chest x-ray, which should be done on all trauma patients.

10. What is the most important blood test to be done in a trauma situation?

    a. Blood alcohol testing

    b. Hematocrit

    c. Type and crossmatch

    d. Arterial blood gases

Answer: c. The most helpful and essential blood test performed in trauma situations is the type and crossmatch, which may be necessary when blood products are indicated.

Chapter 12: Wound and Laceration Repair

The treatment of skin wounds includes mainly the treatment of lacerations, abrasions, and puncture wounds—each of which are treated slightly differently. These are extremely common skin problems affecting nearly everyone at some point in their lives. The goal of the emergency medical physician or dermatologist is to determine what kind of wound the patient has and to use the proper protocols for each of these skin wounds. The focus of this chapter is on the management of wounds and the specific techniques used in emergency laceration repair.

Evaluating a Wound

As soon as the patient presents with a laceration, it should be treated with direct pressure used to control the bleeding. A history of the problem should be obtained, the tetanus status should be obtained, and personal health history for things like diabetes, immunodeficiency states, and HIV should be evaluated. Allergies to latex, antibiotic, local anesthesia, and tape should be asked about.

The wound should be explored to look for foreign bodies and the presence of an injury to parts of the body not simply skin and soft tissue, such as tendons, muscles, bone, blood vessels, ligaments, or nerves. The neurovascular status of the wound should be looked at to make sure there isn't any damage to large vessels or nerves. Any laceration that has ongoing bleeding, exposure of underlying tissue, or are a cosmetic problem need suturing but wounds that don't have these qualities may not necessarily need suturing.

The main goals of laceration repair are to obtain hemostasis, decrease the infection rate, restore physiological functioning, and have better cosmesis of the wound. The time since the injury determines whether or not the wound can be repaired primarily as well as the extent and location of the wound. A surgical consultation should be considered for deep hand or foot wounds, full thickness wounds of the ear, lip, or eyelid, lacerations involving structures other than skin and soft tissue, deep penetrating wounds, crush injuries, wounds where cosmesis is particularly important, and contaminated wound requiring drainage.

Laceration Repair

Before repairing a wound, it should be copiously irrigated with tap water or normal saline. This decreases the bacterial content of a wound and prevents infection after the repair. Warmed irrigating solutions are more comfortable but are not absolutely necessary. No soap, iodine solutions, or hydrogen peroxide should be used as irrigating agents because of their irritation potential. A 30- to 60-ml syringe with a large-bore needle or catheter should be used for irrigation at a moderately-high pressure. Forceps should be used to remove foreign material and a scissors or scalpel should be used to remove devitalized tissue. Any foreign body near a possibly lacerated joint, blood vessel, or nerve should be carefully removed as removal can further damage the structure. The hair should not be shaved but should instead be clipped around the wound. The eyebrows should never be shaved or clipped as the repair depends on the correct positioning of the lacerated ends near the brow hair.

There are many options for skin laceration repair, including skin-closure tapes, staples, tissue adhesives, internal (dissolvable) sutures, and external (non-dissolvable) sutures. It is important to be familiar with all of these techniques because you may be using any one of these techniques in the repair of a laceration, depending on the clinical situation, location of the laceration, and patient preference.

The main things in the recommendations for performing laceration care include the following:

- Either saline or tap water can be used to irrigate the wound, and both hydrogen peroxide and povidone-iodine should be avoided as they are irritating to the skin.

- A local anesthetic, if necessary, should be given slowly to avoid the sting of the injection. Buffering or warming the solution will also decrease the injection site pain.

- The preferred method of caring for a laceration is the application of sutures.

- Tissue adhesion techniques have shown to have similar cosmetic results to suturing, particularly when used on the scalp.

- Antibiotic ointment and the use of petrolatum jelly applied to the wound will provide the same protection against infection.

The evaluation should include a visual inspection to see if the laceration involves muscle, fascia, tendon, bone, or just soft tissue and skin. The neurovascular status of the patient should be assessed prior to repairing the laceration. Functional status of the affected area and areas distal to the wound should be a part of the evaluation.

Any laceration that is actively bleeding or exposes underlying connective tissue needs repair, although wounds on the hand or scalp that aren't bleeding, are superficial and less than two centimeters in total length may be managed with antibacterial ointment alone without suturing.

The main goals of doing a laceration repair are to minimize infection, achieve homeostasis, and restore function to the affected body part. Exactly how a given laceration is repaired depends on the provider's skill, the time since the injury, and the type of available materials to perform the repair.

Exactly when a laceration is to be repaired depends on its location, the origin of the laceration, the degree of contamination, the age of the patient, and the health of the patient. In general, non-contaminated wounds can be successfully sutured up to twelve hours after the injury. Clean lacerations of highly-vascularized tissue can be repaired up to twenty-four hours after the laceration occurred. Some wounds can be packed for a few days before closing them secondarily if it doesn't become infected in the interim.

Any wound, especially one that might have a foreign body or bacterial organisms, should be copiously irrigated with either tap water or normal saline. Warming the irrigant will be more comfortable for the victim and things like povidone-iodine, detergents, and hydrogen peroxide shouldn't be used as they are toxic to the necessary fibroblasts in the area of the wound. All visible foreign body matter should be removed through irrigation or manual removal, using forceps. All devitalized tissue should be sharply debrided to decrease the infection risk. Any hair near the wound should be clipped for better exposure. Shaving of the skin is not recommended, as it is irritating to the skin and will contaminate the wound.

Anesthesia for Wound Repair

Local anesthesia involves 1 percent lidocaine or 0.25 percent bupivacaine. Large wounds, especially those of the extremities, need a regional block. Epinephrine should not be added to the anesthetic if the wound is in an area with end arterioles, including the earlobes, penis, nose, toes and fingers. Smaller needles with warmed or buffered solution will decrease the risk of injection pain. Buffering can be done by adding 8.4 percent sodium bicarbonate (1 milliliter per 10 milliliters of lidocaine solution).

Remember that EMLA (a topical anesthetic containing lidocaine and prilocaine cream) can be used in children or in those who are particularly afraid of injections. It needs to be applied with an occlusive dressing and kept on the wound for up to four hours before doing the repair. Highly-vascular areas need less time to have effectiveness of this technique.

Repair Techniques

As mentioned, options include skin-closure tape, staples, adhesives, and sutures. Wounds that need a multi-layer closure should have suture repair as should wounds over joints and wounds in areas of the body with a thick dermis. Low tension areas and lacerations in children should be considered for closure with a tissue adhesive.

Deep lacerations need repair with absorbable suture to cover the repair of the internal layers with non-absorbable suture used to close the skin. This approach will have better cosmesis, better functional outcome, and will decrease the risk of developing a wound hematoma. Deep layer closure puts less tension on the skin after the repair.

Absorbable sutures for internal repair include polyglycolic acid (Dexon), poliglecaprone 25 (Monocryl), and polyglactin 910 (Vicryl). They are used for deeper closures of muscle and connective tissue as they dissolve in the body within 4-8 weeks. The rate of dehiscence, poor cosmetic result, and rate of infection are the same whether absorbable sutures are used or not.

Nylon-type suture, such as Prolene is used to close the skin. This is non-absorbable and must be removed within 7-10 days after placing the sutures. The use of silk for this purpose is not recommended because there is a great deal of tissue reactivity, with an increased risk of scarring and infection. The finest suture that will still hold the wound together should be used—anywhere from 3-0 Prolene to 6-0 Prolene 3-0 to 4-0 is used when tension an issue, while 4-0 to 5-0 is used on the extremities and trunk in wounds not under tension. 5-0 to 6-0 Prolene sutures are often used on the face.

Methods of suturing include using interrupted closure (multiple tied-off sutures), running closure (with one long strand entering and exiting the skin at different intervals, and subcuticular closure (which requires absorbable suture). Always pierce the skin at a ninety-degree angle and then, with twist of the wrist, bring the curved needle around so that it exits the opposite side at a ninety-degree angle. This allows for eversion of the skin edges and a better cosmetic outcome when it heals. Suturing should start in the middle of the wound and should work outward in a symmetric fashion.

A horizontal mattress suture technique is often used for the closure of high tension wounds or gaping wounds. It is effective because it spreads the tension along the wound's edge. The vertical mattress technique is used when the wound edges need everting in parts of the body that tend to easily invert, such as the back of the neck or a concave surface. Subcuticular sutures cannot be seen from the outside and utilize absorbable suture for the best cosmetic result in facial or other highly-exposed areas.

Tissue adhesives, such as Dermabond, which is 2-octylcyanoacrylate, work in some cases. The cosmetic result, dehiscence rate, and infection risk are the same as with sutures but they have the advantage of being much quicker to apply and, and the fact that they don't require anesthesia is another advantage, especially for children. They do cost more to use than sutures and can't be used in high tension wounds but are great for the face and for very small lacerations. They shouldn't be used if the patient is immunosuppressed or has a condition very much associated with poor wound healing, like diabetes mellitus.

A little-known technique for the scalp includes the hair apposition technique. No suturing is done and hair on either side of the laceration are twisted together and affixed with tissue adhesive. The hair acts as "suture" to approximate the scalp wound. The hair should be at least three inches long and the laceration should be less than ten centimeters in total length.

Staples and Steri-strips can be used to repair many lacerations. Surgical staples are recommended for thick-skinned lesions, such as the trunk, extremities, and scalp. Don't use staples on the hands, feet, neck, or face. Steri-strips are good for low tension, short lacerations but, unless they are well-applied, they can result in wound dehiscence. They strongly rely on the patient's willingness to keep them on until the laceration has completely healed.

Stainless steel staples can be used for thick skinned-skinned areas such as the scalp, trunk, and extremities but never on the hands, feet, neck, and face. Staples should be avoided on the scalp if an MRI or CT scan of the head is believed to be necessary. They work best for achieving quick hemostasis in uncooperative patients, such as those who are intoxicated or children. They are good for multiple trauma patients with many wounds.

Tetanus Prophylaxis Recommendations

Any laceration patient should be asked about their tetanus status. If the patient has an unknown status or has less than three doses in their life time, they should receive TDAP or TD, which Tetanus Immune Globulin given for dirty or unclean wounds. Anyone who has had more than three doses of tetanus toxoid in the past and who has the last dose was within ten years, does not need to have a tetanus booster shot.

Suture Removal Timing

The removal of the sutures depends on where the laceration was located and sometimes on the depth and other wound factors. In general, however, the following guidelines for suture removal should be adhered to:

- **Face**—three to five days

- **Scalp**—seven to ten days

- **Arms**—seven to ten days

- **Trunk**—seven to ten days

- **Legs**—ten to fourteen days

Care of Abrasions

Injures like road rash and abrasions are very common sports-related injuries. These are injures caused by friction of the skin against a rough surface, which causes layers of the skin to come off. Sometimes just the upper layer is taken of (the epidermis), while deeper abrasions will affect the next layer of skin (the dermis). Motorcyclists and cyclists are especially prone to getting rod rash. They tend not to bleed much but are very painful as many nerve endings have been disrupted.

In treating an abrasion or road rash, the area should be cleansed with mild soap and water. If a mild antiseptic soap is available, this would be preferable. Antibiotic ointment and a dry dressing are applied next. It is crucial to remove the debris and dirt from the abrasion in order to prevent infection. A bio-occlusive dressing or semipermeable dressing, like Tegaderm, are good choices for dressings.

Care of Puncture Wounds

Lacerations and puncture wounds may look the same with brief observation. To make the differential diagnosis, it takes gently probing the wound to evaluate it for its depth. If it is deep enough to have possibly endangered internal organs, a more thorough evaluation needs to be undertaken.

Puncture wounds can come from many things. Many animal bites are puncture wounds; all bullet wounds are puncture wounds; and all impaled objects are puncture wounds. Puncture wounds don't have to have a specific depth or size. It basically has to be somewhat deeper than it is long, with an area of deep tissue involvement and possible deeper organ involvement.

The goal of treating puncture wounds is to stop the bleeding using direct pressure on the wound or on arteriovenous pressure points for about fifteen minutes. The puncture wound should then be washed with mild cleanser and water and covered. Puncture wounds, in general, have a high infection rate. Patients need to have a tetanus toxoid injection if they aren't current and the wound is best left open to drain as it heals.

Key Takeaways

- Lacerations require a thorough history as to the mechanism of injury, the patient's tetanus status, allergies, and relevant past medical history.

- Lacerations should be irrigated with water or saline under moderate pressure.

- Laceration repair involves internal (dissolvable) sutures and external (removeable sutures).

- Care of puncture wounds and abrasions depend on the location and depth of the injuries.

Quiz

1. Which type of wound would most likely lead to tetanus?

   a. Superficial laceration of the scalp

   b. Puncture wound of the hand

   c. Abrasion of the shoulder

   d. Deep laceration of the lip

Answer: b. A puncture wound on the hand would have the greatest chance of leading to tetanus as it is on the hand and is a deep wound, which promotes the growth of Clostridium tetani.

2. Which wound would likely need a tetanus booster?

   a. Burn to the trunk

   b. Corneal abrasion

   c. Laceration on the scalp

   d. All of the above

Answer: d. All of the above wounds are prone to tetanus, with a need for a tetanus shot if the patient has not already had one/is already covered with the right number of prior injections.

3. What is recommended to be applied to a laceration or abrasion after cleansing and treating?

   a. Bactroban ointment

   b. Petroleum jelly

   c. Hydrocortisone cream

   d. Dry gauze dressing

Answer: a. While petroleum jelly can provide as good an antibacterial effect when compared to Bactroban in laceration treatment, it is preferred over petroleum jelly for the treatment of abrasions.

4. What type of suture material is used to repair the outer layer of skin in a laceration?

   a. Vicryl

   b. Prolene

   c. Dexon

   d. Monocryl

Answer: b. Nylon or Prolene is used to close the skin in lacerations, with the other types of sutures being commonly used in the subcutaneous layers and not the skin.

5. What is a not a good option for treating a laceration of the face?

   a. Steri-Strip closure

   b. Prolene closure

   c. Staple closure

   d. Tissue adhesive closure

Answer: c. A staple closure is not appropriate for the face because it offers the least in cosmesis when closing the wound.

6. What is the main advantage of doing a subcuticular closure of a wound?

a. Better cosmesis

b. Decreased wound infection

c. Decreased wound inflammation

d. Faster repair time

Answer: a. A subcuticular closure often takes longer but, because there are no visible suture marks, there tends to be better cosmesis of these wounds.

7. Why should silk sutures not be used for the skin?

   a. It causes increased scarring and tissue reaction.

   b. It increases the infection risk.

   c. It is not strong enough for the skin.

   d. It can be used for subcutaneous sutures but not for skin sutures.

Answer: a. Silk should not be used for subcutaneous or surface sutures because it causes increased tissue reaction and scarring.

8. What type of suture would be used to repair an external lip laceration?

   a. 3-0 Prolene

   b. 4-0 Prolene

   c. 5-0 Prolene

   d. 6-0 Prolene

Answer: d. The best suture size for the face and lips would be the smallest size, which is 6-0 Prolene. This will lead to the best cosmesis.

9. You are repairing a high tension wound over an extensor surface. What would be the most appropriate repair technique?

   a. Steri-Strips

   b. Horizontal mattress sutures

   c. Subcuticular repair

   d. Tissue adhesive repair

Answer: b. A high tension wound over an extensor surface needs strong suturing, that includes a horizontal mattress repair.

10. When should sutures placed in the face be removed in most cases?

   a. 3-5 days

   b. 5-7 days

c. 7-10 days

d. 10-14 days

Answer: a. Wounds of the face should have the sutures removed at about 3-5 days after laceration repair with sutures.

Chapter 13: Psychiatric Emergencies

This chapter involves the care and management of psychiatric emergencies. A psychiatric emergency can be defined as any situation in which the healthcare provider confronts a situation in which the patient cannot stop acting on compulsions to harm themselves or another person. The patient may present with full awareness of the impact of their desired behavior but more often than not, they present with a lack of judgment and insight into what might happen should they follow through on their compulsion.

Definition of a Psychiatric Emergency

Patients in a psychiatric emergency may be psychotic, extremely depressed, or manic. The patient, even if they are aware of what might happen if they do the behavior they are suggesting, might still be determined to perform the behavior in spite of obvious risks. Many patients in a psychiatric emergency do not present themselves but are brought to the attention of the healthcare provider by bystanders, family members, friends, police officers, or other community members associated with the patient.

The psychiatric emergency encountered by the healthcare worker can be defined as "aggression" and can include suicidal ideation, homicidal ideation, or thoughts of other violence against another. These, while the intended target is different, are basically the same phenomenon—that of harm intended toward the physical body of oneself or another person.

In dealing with these types of emergencies, all threats made by the patient, regardless of their intent, should be taken very seriously and should not be written off as the ramblings of a psychotic, depressed, or manic patient. Emergent action is required; any underreaction might lead to disastrous consequences. Overreaction, on the other hand, can be frustrating to all parties involved but is worth the risk of unintentionally and unwittingly allowing the patient to follow through on their intentions.

It is important to remember that all psychiatric emergencies fall on a continuum. The mild end of the continuum is the thought of doing a harmful act, while the severe end of the spectrum is already attempting but unsuccessfully completing the intended act. There is a gray area in between and it is up to the provider to make the call as to whether the thought is fleeting and not an intention or whether thought is leading up to an intended act. This is why it is important to ask about things like whether or not the patient has a plan directed at their ideation and whether or not the plan is a feasible one that the patient is capable of carrying out.

Risk Factors for Completed Aggression

There are numerous risk factors for having completed aggressive compulsions, which make the patient's ideation more likely to evolve into an aggressive behavior. These include the following:

- Having a homicidal or suicidal plan that is feasible for the patient to carry out.

- Having a past history of homicidal or suicidal behavior, including a past history of suicide attempts or a criminal history associated with aggression.

- Havin a homicidal or suicidal plan that is truly a lethal one as opposed to something that won't likely really lead to harm to the patient or another person.

- Having any one of the following psychiatric diagnoses: Antisocial or borderline personality disorder, combined Axis I and Axis II disorders, postpartum psychosis, substance withdrawal, substance use disorders (especially PCP, amphetamines, and cocaine), using or withdrawing from alcohol, anorexia nervosa, schizophrenia, bipolar disorder, or major depressive disorder.

- Having any of the following physical conditions: Pain syndrome, lupus, chronic renal failure (on dialysis), COPD, HIV/AIDS, cancer of any kind, seizure disorder of any kind, brain injury, Huntington's disease, or multiple sclerosis.

- Having a severe lack of social support in the family or in the community.

- Being recently unemployed and having a decrease in socioeconomic status.

- Being the perpetrator or victim in a domestic violence situation.

- Having a recent and significant life stressor.

- Having a past history of childhood physical or sexual abuse.

- Having a positive family history of mental disorders, substance use disorders, homicide, or suicide.

- Showing evidence of narcissism, poor self-esteem, psychological pain or turmoil, humiliation or shame, panic attacks, sever anxiety, or extreme hopelessness.

- Being or showing evidence of impulsiveness.

- Being agitated.

- Having marked polarization of thinking, tunnel vision, loss of normal executive functioning, or showing evidence of lack of reasoning.

- Being of the male gender.

- Being unmarried through divorce, separation, widowhood, or never marrying.

- Being an adolescent (male or female).

- Being either bisexual or homosexual/lesbian.

- Having access to firearms or other weapons, or having access to drugs that might be implicated in an overdose situation.

- Being currently intoxicated with something that impairs executive function and impulsivity.

- Having no psychotherapist or a poor relationship the patient's psychotherapist.

Factors related to Prevalence

Any homicidal ideation related to the workplace should be taken seriously, particularly if the patient was just fired or became recently unemployed. Homicidal activity in the workplace is, however, extremely uncommon, affecting about 1 out of 100,000 employed persons. Most commonly, the events of aggression have been related to firearms and the shooting was often randomly directed at the workplace. Access to firearms should be assessed when dealing with this type of ideation. Drug use is also highly associated with workplace violence.

While the actual annual incidence of suicide is only about 11 completed suicides out of 100,000 people and the estimated lifetime risk of suicide in the average person is just 0.7 percent, this is definitely not the case with patients who have a mood disorder or schizophrenia. Patients with any type of mood disorder have about a 15 percent lifetime risk of completed suicide and patients who have attempted suicide in the past have a 25 percent chance of successfully completing suicide so this should be asked about in the history of the patient. For patients with schizophrenia, the lifetime risk of completed suicide is about six percent.

Statistically, women make more suicide attempts than men but men have a higher risk of completed suicide, mainly because they use more violent methods of attempting suicide, such as hanging oneself, jumping from a high place, and shooting oneself. The actual death rate from suicide is highest in men aged 40-44 years, although the completed suicide rate of men older than 65 years of age is also very high at about 60 completed suicides out of 100,000 people. Suicide is also common in the 14-25-year-old age group, being the third leading cause of death in this population.

It is important to remember that aggressive acts, whether they be directed at oneself or another person, ultimately stem from feelings of anger, fear, hopelessness, and frustration, even though those feelings might be irrational or only perceived by the patient himself. The taking of any drug or chemical that intensifies these feelings only increases the risk that the ideation will turn in to a completed act of aggression.

Signs and Symptoms of a Psychiatric Emergency

Sometimes it just takes the healthcare provider to recognize in themselves a sense of irritability, fear, or discomfort that is directly coming from the interaction with the patient. This can be a barometer toward detecting whether or not to be concerned about sending the patient back out into the community.

There are certain patient characteristics that might lead the provider to take the patient's ideation or threats more seriously. Patients with wounds or scars on their body suggest that they have been in violent situations in the past and have a greater propensity to be in this type of situation in the present. Those with primitive tattoos suggest impulsivity and a connection to darker elements in society. Abnormal pupil size and reactivity indicate that the patient may be suffering the effects of an intoxicating drug that is impairing their judgment.

Patients that seem determined, with a fixed gaze and flat affect, are at a greater risk of actually following through on their ideation. The use of threatening or profane speech suggests a propensity toward violence and those with obviously increased skeletal muscle tension have a greater chance of being violent toward themselves or others. The presence of pacing or hyperactivity suggests a tendency toward violent behaviors. Being violent during the examination or acting in threatening ways during the examination is a sign that the patient might follow through on their aggressive ideation.

Intervention in a Psychiatric Emergency

The first goal in intervention is attempting to build rapport with the patient so they can be more honest with you regarding their intentions. If this isn't possible, the provider should involve other people in the patient's life in order to obtain collaborating information and to try to see if others can share in the responsibility and safety of the patient and any others the violent ideation is directed toward. If psychosis is part of the evaluation, a medical clearance should be performed to make sure the patient doesn't have an underlying medical reason for being psychotic.

Upon deciding that the patient is at risk for aggressive self-directed or other-directed behavior, security might have to become involved or the police might have to be contacted. Arrangements must be made to house the patient in a locked psychiatric ward if their behavior and ideation has been deemed purely psychiatric in nature. In some cases, the provider should make the decision to contact the person being threatened by the patient in order to make sure they are sufficiently warned of the threat against them.

If the patient presents to the evaluation with a weapon or other means of harming themselves or others, rapport should be established to the greatest degree possible before asking the patient if they would be willing to give up control of the dangerous implement. This will immediately decrease the impending threat but indicates that the patient probably has a serious intent toward aggression and should be housed in a safe place until the threat has passed. Allowing the patient to relinquish the control over the weapon voluntarily is much safer than aggressively trying to take control of the object.

The healthcare provider is himself at risk of violence in cases of an individual who expresses aggression toward others. In such situations, the provider should see the patient with the help of security personnel and should never see the patient in a situation where the patient and provider are isolated from help in case the patient should become acutely violent.

Medications used to Treat the Aggressive Psychotic Patient

The aggressive psychotic patient may need medical intervention; this can control their psychosis and in particular can control their delusions, which put them at risk for carrying out their aggressive intent. Patients already on antipsychotic medications are still candidates for medical therapy to control aggression. The first line agent for this type of emergency is a neuroleptic medication.

There are two classes of antipsychotic medications that can be helpful in an acute psychosis situation. The newer atypical antipsychotic agents include clozapine, olanzapine, quetiapine, and risperidone. The older agents can also be helpful and include chlorpromazine, fluphenazine, haloperidol, thioridazine, and thiothixene (among others). Any of these medications can be helpful in an acute setting. There are fewer side effects with the atypical antipsychotics, however.

Relief of psychosis can happen within a few hours after taking the drug. Multiple antipsychotic drugs can be used. There is no benefit over using injectable medications versus oral medications in an acute setting. It is not acceptable is simply give an antipsychotic medication and discharge the patient. These patients need in-hospital stabilization before discharge.

Treatment of the Suicidal Patient

The suicidal patient may present by themselves but more often presents with a concerned loved one to whom they have confided there is suicidal intent. All suicidal ideation should be taken seriously with a hospital admission. It is not satisfactory to send them home on antidepressant medications or to send them home with a loved one who cannot guarantee their safety.

The highest risk patients are those who have a suicidal plan and especially those with a lethal plan. Patients who live alone and have little social support also are at high risk. Any patient with a chronic pain condition or chronic illness has a statistically higher risk of carrying out a suicidal plan. The goal is to be proactive and arrange for their emergent admission where long-term follow-up, the starting of medical therapy, and an improvement in psychosocial situation can be carried out.

The diagnoses that place the person at the greatest risk for suicide include major depression, schizophrenia, bipolar disorder, and substance use disorder. The diagnosis most associated with attempted or completed suicide is major depression.

Key Takeaways

- A psychiatric emergency can involve an aggression toward oneself or to another person.

- Men have a higher rate of completed suicide when compared to women.

- People under the influence of drugs or alcohol have poor judgment, which makes them a psychiatric emergency risk.

- Major depression carries the highest risk of completed suicide.

Quiz

1. A patient in a psychiatric emergency is least likely to have what type of psychiatric problem?

   a. Mania

   b. Psychosis

   c. Depression

   d. Somatization

Answer: d. Patients with mania, psychosis, and depression are most likely to present with a psychiatric emergency, while patients with somatization are least likely to present in an emergency situation.

2. Which scenario is least likely to occur with regard to a psychiatric emergency?

   a. The patient is brought into the emergency room by the police.

   b. The patient presents with the complaint of homicidal ideation.

   c. Family members become concerned about the patient's degree of suicidal ideation.

   d. A psychiatrist refers the patient to the emergency department because of severe psychosis and an inability to care for himself.

Answer: b. Patients with these types of psychiatric emergencies are not likely to present themselves with their emergency situation but are brought by police, family members, friends, or healthcare workers.

3. What global term best defined the phenomenon happening with a patient who has a psychiatric emergency?

   a. Self-harm behaviors

   b. Suicidal ideation

   c. Aggression

   d. Homicidal ideation

Answer: c. All forms of psychiatric emergencies involve aggression, which may be directed at the self or at others. The other terms are not all-inclusive when it comes to a psychiatric emergency.

4. What factor makes a suicide by a male more likely to succeed when compared to women?

   a. They have a decreased rate of being treated for depression.

   b. They have a tendency toward more lethal suicidal plans.

   c. They have a higher risk of having psychotic depression.

   d. They are more likely to have a suicidal action when suffering from psychosis.

Answer: b. The male suicide act is more likely to be completed when compared to a female suicide act because they often have a more lethal suicide plan when compared to women.

5. Which personality disorder is more likely to be associated with a suicidal plan?

   a. Schizoid personality disorder

   b. Dependent personality disorder

   c. Antisocial personality disorder

   d. Histrionic personality disorder

Answer: c. Patients with antisocial or borderline personality disorder are more prone to a suicidal ideation and a completed suicidal plan.

6. In a patient who has aggressive or homicidal intent related to the workplace, what plan is more likely to be carried out?

   a. The use of firearms against the workplace without a specific person in mind.

   b. The intent to cause an accident regarding one's boss.

   c. The intent to harm specific people in the workplace.

   d. The intent to commit suicide after killing someone in the workplace.

Answer: a. While workplace homicide is rare, anyone with the intent to use firearms to kill anyone at the workplace is the most commonly-listed ideation. Access to firearms should be addressed in these situations.

7. What is the mainstay of treatment for the suicidal patient?

   a. Antipsychotic medications to control suicidal delusions

   b. Antidepressant medications to control depressive symptoms

   c. Inpatient admission to a locked psychiatric unit

   d. Twenty-four-hour follow-up with a mental health professional for therapeutic intervention

Answer: c. Patients with suicidal ideation need an inpatient admission to a locked psychiatric unit, regardless of their ideation. It is not acceptable to discharge them, even if they are under the care of a responsible person.

8. Which patient has the least risk of carrying out a completed suicide when presenting to the emergency department with suicidal ideation?

   a. The patient who is already taking an antidepressant

   b. The patient with a lethal suicidal plan

   c. The patient with no social support

   d. The patient with a chronic illness or pain condition

Answer: a. All of the above patients have a high risk of completing suicide. The patient already on an antidepressant has no greater risk when compared to the other choices.

9. Which mental illness carries the greatest risk for attempted and completed suicide?

   a. Schizophrenia

   b. Bipolar disorder

   c. Major depression

   d. Substance use disorder

Answer: c. The patient with major depression has the greatest risk for attempted and completed suicide. The others are of a greater than average risk but do not have as high a risk as major depression.

10. When would the least likely situation be that would place the emergency room provider at risk for injury?

   a. In a patient who is acutely intoxicated.

   b. In a patient who is agitated during the examination.

   c. In a patient who throws something during the evaluation.

   d. In a patient who says he is having auditory hallucinations.

Answer: d. All of the above patients pose a risk to the healthcare provider but the patient having hallucinations carries the least risk toward harming the provider evaluating them.

Chapter 14: Toxicology in the Emergency Setting

The study of toxicology involves both the study of toxic medications that are not normally toxic under typical situations but become toxic in high doses. It also involves the study of those things that are always toxic to the body. There are some things that are toxic to the kidneys, toxic to the heart, toxic to the lungs, toxic to a growing fetus, or toxic to the ears. All of these things will be covered in this chapter.

Toxic Exposures

Many organic and inorganic chemicals can be toxic to the human body. The exact toxicity of a chemical depends on the class the chemical belongs in. Researchers have identified certain "toxic syndromes" that are also called "toxidromes". A toxidrome represents a certain set of health effects caused by a particular class of chemical. Each toxidrome is a specific set of toxic effects that provide a fingerprint unique to the class of toxins. Toxidromes are worth memorizing because all chemical agents of a given toxidrome are treated roughly the same in an emergency setting.

The following are some toxidromes you should memorize as they have classic findings on presentation:

- **Anticholinergic Toxidrome.** This class of toxins leads to a decreased stimulation of the cholinergic receptors (muscarinic receptors) with clinical findings that include the presence of pupillary dilation (mydriasis), dry skin with an absence of sweating, increased body temperature, hallucinations, and other mental status changes.

- **Anticoagulant Toxidrome.** This class of toxins involves altering the coagulability of the blood so that there is excessive or abnormal bleeding episodes. This can present to the emergency room with the clinical picture of excessive bruising, bleeding from the stomach, bleeding from the respiratory mucous membranes, bladder bleeding, intestinal bleeding, and bleeding from internal locations (such as subdural bleeding, other intracranial bleeding, or retroperitoneal bleeding.

- **Solvents, Anesthetics, and Sedatives Toxidrome.** Exposure to these chemicals and toxic substances leads to CNS depression and decreased level of consciousness that may or may not lead to a coma. Respirations are depressed by these toxins and some people have difficulty walking and standing, with a prominence of ataxia when trying to walk.

- Convulsant Toxidrome. This involves an overall excitation of the CNS with either antagonism of the (calming) GABA system or agonism of the (excitatory) glutamate system, leading to prolonged seizures. Convulsants can be drugs or toxic substances.

- **Cholinergic Toxidrome.** This is also called pesticide or nerve agent syndrome. It involves an overstimulation of the cholinergic receptors, particularly in the end organs of the nervous system. It starts with activation of the target organs and then leads to fatigue of these organs. Pupils tend to be pinpoint and people exposed to these agents will often have seizures, twitching, wheezing, and excessive secretions from nearly all secretory organs (increased salivation, tearing, vomiting, incontinence, sweating, and bronchial secretions).

- **Irritant/Corrosive Toxidrome.** There are immediate effects upon touching one of these toxins that range from minor irritation of any skin exposed to the toxin, irritation of mucous membranes, irritation of the GI tract, or irritation of the lungs. This can lead to wheezing, coughing, and respiratory distress, or to severe involvement of the GI tract that lead to absorption of the toxin, which can go on to cause systemic toxicity.

- **Knockdown Toxidrome.** This is a unique toxidrome that specifically involves a disruption in the cellular oxygen delivery to the peripheral tissues secondary to displacement of oxygen by other gases (carbon monoxide or methemoglobin inducers), hemoglobinopathies, or asphyxia that leads to an impairment of either the oxygen transport by the red blood cell or an impairment of the peripheral tissue's ability to make use of oxygen. Toxins of this class include mitochondrial metabolism inhibitors (including cyanide). Common symptoms associated with this toxidrome include having an altered state of consciousness, lightheadedness or fatigue, progressing to seizures and coma. There is toxicity to the heart as well, which can lead to sudden cardiac death.

- **Opioid Toxidrome.** This involves a toxin or drug that is agonistic to the opioid receptors, leading to pinpoint pupils, respiratory depression, and central nervous system depression. The effects mimic the body's normal reaction to opioid receptor excitability but to an excessive degree, leading to toxicity and adverse side effects.

- **Sympathomimetic Toxidrome.** This involves a toxin that mimics activation of the sympathetic nervous system. It induces an excess of catecholamines and CNS excitation, which ultimately leads to panic, confusion, increased respirations, increased pulse, and increased blood pressure.

Emergency Treatment of a Toxic Exposure

When a patient arrives at the emergency department, often the exact chemical is not known so it is doubly important to recognize exactly what toxidrome is being represented as this provides a gauge to how the patient is treated.

In evaluating the patient with a possible toxic exposure, it takes just a few simple observations, including pupil size and reactivity, mental status, vital signs, irritation of the mucous membranes, evaluation of lung sounds, and evaluation of the skin for color, moisture, and chemical burns. The specific group of symptoms needs to be identified before the patient progresses to cardiac arrest, prolonged seizures, or coma. After the life-threatening crisis has been overcome and the patient is stable, more information about the exact nature of the exposure and other details can be obtained. In this case, the drug is identified as belonging to a certain toxidrome and the treatment is directed at the toxidrome.

The route of the exposure determines the level of toxicity and the type of toxicity experienced by the patient. For example, consider the condition of inhalation exposure. This includes any exposure to toxic vapors, gases, airborne powders, or aerosolized liquids. Each of these represents an inhalation risk. Inhalation of irritating gases attack the watery component of the respiratory mucosa and the eyes, causing burning eye pain, burning chest pain, irritation of the bronchial tree, and increased secretions wherever the toxin came in contact with the body.

Inhalation can cause a rapid entry of the toxin into the system via the respiratory tract, causing effects that are not located close to the site of entry. An example of this type of exposure is being exposed to hydrogen cyanide gas. The portal of entry is the respiratory tract but the symptoms come from entry into the system, causing seizures, cardiac arrhythmias, loss of consciousness, hypotension, and possible sudden death within minutes following the exposure.

Skin or dermal exposure involves the direct contact of a toxic chemical that absorbs through the skin, causing systemic findings outside of the range of the actual site of exposure. An example of a toxin that does this is an organophosphate insecticide exposure. It rapidly penetrates the skin (because it is fat-soluble) and gets into the system. Skin exposure will eventually cause symptoms; however, there is often a delayed reaction when compared to exposure via the lungs.

It is a good idea to get an estimate of the dose of the toxin the patient came in contact with. The dose is the total amount of the toxin absorbed by whatever means during the exposure. The dose depends both on the concentration of the chemical and the contact time (duration of exposure). Most chemicals cause a predictable effect based on the dose the patient got. Alcohol is an example of this. Certain doses can predictably yield a specific systemic response that might include an alteration of consciousness (low doses or mild inebriation), loss of coordination (moderate inebriation), and respiratory arrest/coma (severe inebriation).

The duration of the exposure affects the dose the patient receives. Long durations of exposure to higher concentrations of toxin lead to more severe effects on the body when compared to lower concentrations and/or decreased duration of exposure. For example, if an acid is applied to the skin, it takes a while for it to penetrate the skin so that, if it is washed off before penetrating the skin, the actual internal damage will be minimal. With inhalations, the longer the breathing time of the toxin, the greater the effect on the body the toxin will have.

Toxicology Testing in the Emergency Room

Rapid toxicology testing is often done in the emergency department to evaluate a patient with a possible toxic exposure or to determine what illicit drug the patient is under the influence of. Most toxicology screens of the blood or urine can return within an hour or so at a major hospital and will provide valuable information as to the patient's clinical status.

Toxicology testing is also referred to as a "tox screen". It checks for levels or just the presence of a drug or toxin in the saliva, blood, or urine. There can be various routes of exposure, including inhalation, ingestion, injection, or absorption through the mucous membranes or skin. Tox screens may also involve the testing of stomach contents (such as in an overdose situation) or testing for the presence of a toxin in a person's sweat. It can test for a single drug but more often checks for the presence of multiple drugs/toxins at the same time. A tox screen can include a screen for certain prescription medications, nonprescription medications, illicit substances, vitamins, alcohol, or supplements.

In actuality, it is easier to test the saliva or urine for the presence of a substance, especially when the test does not require an actual level but only needs a "yes" or "no" response. Blood testing is more invasive and will not generally provide a better evaluation of the patient's exposure. Urine testing will detect exposures that occurred days prior to the patient's presentation and can give a more accurate measure of the patient's recent use of illicit substances.

The different purposes of a toxicology test include the following:

- To see if a person's severe or life-threatening symptoms are secondary to a drug overdose or toxic exposure. It must be done within 4 days of ingestion or exposure.

- To test for illicit drug use among workers. This is a common practice among people who work in public safety positions (like airline pilots or bus drivers) or people who work in sensitive jobs, such as childcare workers or healthcare. It is done whenever there is an accident in the workplace for which the worker receives medical attention.

- To check students or other athletes who are injured in a sporting activity or other extracurricular activity. This is not usually a legal issue but may explain their constellation of symptoms.

- To evaluate the drug and alcohol exposure after a motor vehicle accident or other legal incident.

- To check for the presence of the "date rape drug" in cases of sexual assault where the victim reports an altered state of consciousness during the rape or sexual assault.

The vast majority of toxicology tests are qualitative tests. Most tests are of the saliva, urine, or blood but other areas of the body can be assessed in unusual situations. The tests will indicate the presence of the drug above a certain low threshold. If the test is positive for the presence of the drug, a quantitative test can be done. Generally, the only useful quantitative toxicology screen comes from a blood screen versus screening any other body fluid or area. Quantitative testing is especially important in alcohol screening, where the level indicates a certain constellation of expected symptoms.

The results of the test can be "negative" meaning no substances were found in the urine, blood, or saliva. The test can be "normal", meaning that the substance (prescription or nonprescription drug) is found but is found within the therapeutic range. The test can also be abnormal, meaning the levels are too low, above the therapeutic range, or so high that the drug might cause toxicity.

Elevated levels of a substance can be secondary to an intentional or unintentional overdose. It can mean there was a single large ingestion of the substance or a long-term excessive use of the substance. High levels don't always mean that the substance is being taken incorrectly. It could mean that the drug is being absorbed to a greater degree by the person's GI tract or that it isn't being processed successfully by the body, leading to a buildup of the drug.

Some medications can alter the results of a toxicology screen because a drug is mistakenly identified as being a drug of abuse. This is true of certain cough medications, which can be ingested and will mistakenly be identified as a positive opiate screen. Other cough medications contain alcohol so there will be a false positive for alcohol as well.

Urine testing tends to be better than blood testing because small traces of most drugs will show up in the urine much longer than they appear in the blood test. In fact, drug use within five days of testing will generally still show a positive test of the urine, when this is not the case with blood. Saliva tests will show drug use within the past 24 hours.

The one thing that a standard toxicology screen will not detect are substances that are inhaled, such as when a person inhales a household product through "sniffing" in order to get intoxicated. This includes products such as nail polish remover (acetone), glues, cleaning fluids, spray paints, lighter fluids, and other inhaled substances.

The only thing a breath test can accurately measure is the approximate alcohol content in a person's system. No other drugs of abuse or other substances can be picked up by a breath test. Urine or saliva testing is necessary to check for any other drug of abuse.

Central Nervous System Toxicity

One of the more sensitive areas of the body when it comes to toxic exposure includes the nervous system. The nervous system is roughly divided into the central nervous system (CNS) and the peripheral nervous system (PNS). The peripheral nervous system is generally outside the blood-brain barrier but the CNS is inside the blood-brain barrier so it reacts differently to toxins. Some toxins just affect the PNS, while others will just affect the CNS. Organophosphates affect both systems by blocking acetylcholinesterase at the neuronal synapses in both the CNS and PNS.

Unfortunately, the CNS has a poor capacity for regeneration and repair so any damage that occurs tends to be relatively permanent. The brain itself is extremely sensitive to hypoglycemia, toxic exposures, and hypoxia because it has a high degree of energy demands. The CNS effects of drugs can cause four separate things to happen: movement disorders, encephalopathy, seizures, or mental status changes.

CNS toxicity has certain manifestations, depending on which agent is involved and on how much exposure there is likely to be. Toxicity from more than one agent can complicate the picture as different effects on the CNS can occur, which can be either synergistic or additive. They can even act opposite to one another, as is the case with opiate and cocaine ingestion at the same time.

An altered mental status can range from agitation of the individual to a deep coma. Things like delirium and symptoms suggestive of dementia can occur with CNS toxicity from drugs or toxins. People with cocaine toxicity or anticholinergic delirium both can cause sedation or agitation, depending on a number of factors. The excitatory neurotransmitter in the CNS is glutamic acid, while the inhibitory neurotransmitter in the brain is GABA. Neurotransmitters like serotonin and catecholamines can be involved. Sympathomimetic drugs will cause neuronal excitation and agitation. Benzodiazepine withdrawal will also cause agitation secondary to a decrease in neuronal activation of GABA receptors that normally occurs with benzodiazepines.

Agitated patients can present with anything from a slight nervousness to violent behaviors. The excessive excitation of the CNS can be life-threatening. Rhabdomyolysis is a major complication of excessive motor activity secondary to agitation and increased physical activity. This can lead to secondary renal failure as myoglobin builds up in the kidneys. This is an emergency situation requiring possible sedation of the patient to retard their psychomotor agitation.

Delirium and dementia may seem the same but they are distinct diagnoses. Delirium is an acute, organic brain condition with a fluctuating level of impairment, difficulties in maintaining attention, alterations in psychomotor activity, disordered sleep, and altered levels of consciousness. This, while severe, can easily be reversed without sequelae. Dementia is gradual in onset and does not reflect an altered level of consciousness as is seen in dementia. These patients are generally completely alert during the evaluation, which is not the case with delirium. It is also not fluctuating, nor is it reversible.

Delirium is the end result of many toxins. The toxidromes mainly associated with delirium include the sympathomimetic drugs (like amphetamines and cocaine), and the anticholinergic drugs (such as atropine). Other drugs will cause agitation and delirium when withdrawing from the drug. This includes alcohol and benzodiazepines.

The psychedelic drugs and hallucinogens (such as LSD and PCP) will cause perceptual changes, hallucinations, agitation, and delirium as well. There is a heightened perception of reality and distortions in reality that cause vivid hallucinations (usually visual) and a heightened state of arousal.

Certain drugs can cause a decrease in mental status. These include drugs that cause drowsiness, altered level of awareness, and eventual coma. There are different ways to describe an altered state of consciousness in these situations. They include "obtundation", which means a mild to moderate reduction in alertness, "stuporous", which means the patient needs vigorous stimulation to be aroused, and "comatose" meaning that the patient cannot be aroused.

Certain drugs may result in seizures as part of toxicity or withdrawal from the drug. There are a number of drugs that can cause seizures. Some directly cause seizures, while others cause seizures upon withdrawal of the drug:

- Theophylline

- Tricyclic antidepressants
- Opiates
- Organophosphates
- Isoniazid
- Insulin (hypoglycemia)
- Salicylates
- Barbiturate withdrawal
- Ethanol withdrawal
- Lindane

- Cocaine
- Carbon monoxide
- Cyanide
- Amphetamines
- Anticholinergics
- Metaldehyde
- Penicillin
- Bupropion
- Lead
- Lithium

Seizures caused by toxins can happen because of an imbalance between the GABA system and the glutamate system and generally are tonic-clonic (grand mal) seizures. Drugs like tricyclic antidepressants act on the sodium channel (in the neuronal cell membrane) causing depolarization and decreasing the seizure threshold. Cyanide causes seizures by causing hypoxia in the brain. This causes membrane leakage and an increase in neuronal firing. Things that block the adenosine receptors will precipitate seizures. Drugs that do this include caffeine and theophylline.

Other drugs and toxins will cause what is known as "encephalopathy". This is a condition of decreased mental status, personality changes, and a decrease in intellectual capacity. No one knows how encephalopathy happens. Some encephalopathy orignates from non-CNS sources. An example of this is an acetaminophen overdose, which damages the liver to such a degree that it causes hepatic encephalopathy. Carbon tetrachloride does the same thing. Valproic acid toxicity causes encephalopathy by inhibiting the synthesis of free fatty acids, resulting in steatosis of the liver and a buldup of ammonia. High ammonia levels are behind this mechanism and are the basis of the findings seen in hepatic encephalopathy.

Some drugs will cause movement disorders, inlcuding things like drug-induced Parkinsonism and neuroleptic malignant syndrome. Drugs that can cause a movement disorder include the following:

- Trazodone

- SSRIs

- Monoamine oxidase inhibitors (MAOIs)

- Selective serotonin reuptake inhibitors (SSRIs)

Drug-induced Parknsonism will mimic true Parkinson's disease in practically every way. There is dystonia, dyskinesia, akasthesia, and other movement dysfunction. Botulinum toxin can reverse some of the dystonia seen in the disorder. Reserpine can cause improvement in the chorea symptoms (addressing the serotonin and dopamine systems).

Stroke is a result of the direct or indirect effects of certain drugs. Things like amphetamines and cocaine (sympathomimetic drugs) will cause hypertension (and either ishchemic or hemorrhagic strokes). Chronic use of ephedrine will cause an acute intracebral hemorrhage and vasculitis of the CNS. Infarction and hemorrhage can result in death from long-term use of ephedrine. Phenylpropanolamine is also a sympathomimetic drug that can cause intracerebral hemorrhages and stroke.

There are four common things that can be given to correct most states of altered mental status. These are often given routinely when the exact cause of the alteration in mental status is not know as they won't harm the patient if given and can make a difference if certain things are causing the mental status changes. These include dextrose (giving sugar in cases of hypoglycemia), oxygen (to correct hypoxia), naloxone (to reverse opiate intake), and thiamine (to reverse a thiamine deficiency). These will work on most cases of unidentified but treatable altered mental status.

Some drugs will naturally cause CNS sedation or depression. Airway management is crucial in these situations as they often result in the end-finding of respiratory failure. Naloxone should be given if an opiate ingestion is suspected to be the cause of the problem. The goal of this therapy is to restore the patient's respiratory drive and hopefully to avoid having to intubate the patient. The effects of naloxone can last between 45 minutes and 70 minutes, so it may need to be repeated. A continuous infusion may be necessary if the half-life of the opiate ingested is longer than that of naloxone. The maximum dose of naloxone in a single bolus is 10 milligrams.

Other antidotes that can be given include flumazenil, which is given for suspected benzodiazepine overdoses. The downside of doing this is that the patient may have withdrawal symptoms, which can include seizures. It is given intravenously at 0.1 to 0.3 mg IV over 30 seconds, up to a maximum dose of 5 mg. Thiamine is still another antidote used to treat patients with Wernicke's encephalopathy. A total of 100 mg is given intravenously over five minutes and is repeated every 6 hours. This will not harm the patient who is not thiamine-deficient.

Hepatic Toxicity

Toxicity to the liver generally causes "toxic hepatitis". There are several things that can lead to liver damage and toxic hepatitis. These include the following:

- Acetaminophen—chronic heavy use of the drug or use with alcohol can precipitate toxic hepatitis and liver failure.

- Alcohol—heavy drinking that occurs over a long period of time will lead to what is known as "alcoholic hepatitis". Rarely, a binge drinking episode can lead to alcoholic hepatitis.

- Certain presciption mediactions—these include the statin drugs, Augmentin, phenytoin, azathoprine, niacin, anabolic steroids, and ketoconazole.

- Chemicals in the workplace—chemicals in the workplace can cause problems with the liver, incluing carbon tetrachloride, polychlorinated biphenols, paraquat (a herbicide), and vinyl chloride.

Nephrotoxicity

The kidneys are especially vulnerable to toxic exposures and will be damaged by direct toxicity or a change in the electrolyte pattern of the bloodstream. It can be temporary, with brief elevations of the creatinine or BUN. If these are detected early enough and the underlying toxicity is treated, the renal toxicity can possibly be reversed. Nephrotoxicity is basically referred to as kidney toxicity or renal toxicity.

The labwork can more precisely identify a patient as having renal toxicity. There is an elevation in the BUN because of a buildup of nitrogenous wastes in the bloodstream as the kidney can no longer clear them from the system. Creatinine is also elevated as it cannot be cleared by the kidneys after being made as a product of energy metabolism. Normal levels of BUN are 10-25 mg/dL, while normal levels of creatinine are 0.7-1.4 mg/dL.

Certain drugs are particularly known for being nephrotoxic. These include many chemotherapy drugs (cisplatin, methotrexate, and carboplatin), biologic therapies (like interferon-alpha and interleukin-2), certain antibiotics (amphotericin B, vancomycin, and gentamycin), ACE inhibitors, NSAIDs, furosemide, and IV contrast dye.

Lung Toxicity

Lung damage can involve a toxic reaction to certain drugs, particularly certain cancer treatments. It is also referred to as acute pulmonary toxicity. The toxin induces inflammation of the lungs and a reduction in the amount of oxygen that can be taken in by the body, leading to fatigue and shortness of breath. It may be a short-term phenomenon or a long-term and permanent problem. Acute pulmonary toxicity tends to be short-lived, while chronic pulmonary toxicity is referred to as "late pulmonary toxicity".

Inflammation of the lungs is known as pneumonitis. It affects the alveolar lining cells and therefore affects gas exchange int the lungs. This can lead to hypoxia. Fibrosis is more chronic and causes the lungs to stiffen. Fibrosis generally occurs over several months after an episode of pneumonitis. It can be a minimal thing or can become progressive, leading to worsened symptoms over time.

Both radiation therapy and chemotherapy can affect the lungs by forming free oxygen radicals. These are unstable molecules that damage cellular structures. It tends to be worse in the lungs because there is a lot of oxgen in the lungs already. Any chemotherapy drug has the capacity to damage lung tissue. Typical chemotherapy drugs most known to cause lung damage include arsenic trioxide, adarubicin, and bleomycin. Other chemotherapy drugs can cause lung toxicity but to a lesser extent.

Typical lung symptoms of pneumonitis or fibrosis of the lungs include fatigue, shortness of breath with activity, cough, and worsened sypmptoms while lying on one's back. The main treatments for lung toxicity include corticosteroids (to decrease inflammation), oxygen therapy (to improve shortness of breath), narcotics (to relieve shortness of breath), and exercises to improve lung function.

Cardiac Toxicity

Cardiac toxicity can be secondary to prescription drugs, chemotherapy treatments, or illicit substances. They can be abruptly damaging to the heart or slowly cause the heart to fail. They can damage the heart muscle or can disrupt the rhythm system of the heart. Certain heart toxins can be fatal if not treated promptly.

Cardiac toxins include any of the following:

- **Cocaine**—this can cause long-term or short-term problems with the heart by increasing the heart rate and blood presure. It can cause a sudden heart attack or stroke. Chronic use can result in dilated cardiomyopathy and congestive heart failure.

- **Ecstasy or MDMA**—this can damage the heart by causing an arrhythmia of the heart and sometimes sudden cardiac death. Tachycardia can also result from MDMA use.

- **Methylphenidate and amphetamines**—medications used for ADHD (such as these amphetamine drugs) can cause an arrhythmia and sudden death or high blood pressure if taken in excess.

- **Chemotherapy**—certain chemotherapy drugs can cause cardiotoxicity. A typical chemotherapy drug that causes this is doxorubicin, which targets the epidermal growth factor receptor type 2. It causes a weakness of the heart function and palpitations.

- **Chest irradiation**—any high dose irradiation to the heart will cause damage to the heart, increasing the risk of dying from heart disease. This is a particular problem in women who have breast irradiation secondary to breast cancer.

- **CT scan irradiation**—CT scanning traditionally has resulted in higher doses of radiation when compared to regular x-rays, although more recently the trend is to use lower doses of radiation.

- **Erectile dysfunction drugs**—these types of drugs (such as sildenafil) can cause an overburdening of the heart that makes them dangerous to use with patients who have heart problems. Patients who take nitrates for heart problems cannot take erectile dysfunction drugs as a dangerous drop in blood pressure can occur.

- **HIV medications**—the HAART therapy used for HIV patients may damage the heart, leading to higher incidences of atherosclerosis, heart failure, heart attack, and stroke in these patients.

- **Mercury poisoning**—this is an environmental pollutant found mainly in eating fish that contain the substance. Taking in too much mercury can result in arrhythmias, hypertension, and an incease in heart disease risk.

Ototoxicity

Certain drugs and exposures can be ototoxic, meaning they can do damage to the cochlea, the auditory nerve, or the entire vestibular system. The effects can fortunately be temporary in many cases but, in a few cases, the ototoxicity can be permanent. Typical ototoxic drugs include cisplatin, furosemide, genamycin, and aspirin. There are others but these are less likely to be ototoxic.

Typical signs and symptoms of ototoxicity include significant hearing loss, tinnitis, and vertigo. The cochlea is the hearing component of the ear and when it is damaged, hearing loss results. High frequency hearing loss happens first and, after this, it progresses to lower frequencies and total hearing loss. The problem may be unilateal or bilateral. Tinnitus can replace the lost hearing. Damage to the semi-circular canals can affect a person's balance and equilibrium.

When the vestibule and the semi-circular canals get damaged, it can adversely affect the eyes. Patients can have nystagmus or oscillopsia when their ears are damaged. They may have difficulty processing images and they may have lightheadedness, wooziness, and dizziness. The least affected part of the ear with ototoxicity is the actual cranial nerve (CN VIII); however, if it is affected, there is less likely to be a return of normal ear function and the person will have permanent tinnitus, deafness, difficulty walking, and balancing problems.

Teratogens

A teratogen is any substance that can cause a birth defect in a growing fetus. It may be an environmental thing, a street drug, a prescription drug, or alcohol that a woman is exposed to during her pregnancy. It is estimated that about five percent of all birth defects are secondary to a teratogenic exposure. It takes about nine days for the conceptus to get to the uterus and implant into the uterine lining. At about 10-14 days, the teratogen can begin having an effect.

At certain times, specific parts of development are affected by the different teratogens. Closure of the neural tube happens at around four weeks gestation so this is the time when a teratogen can most affect the neural tube closure. Some systems are affected by teratogens throughout the pregnancy, such as the central nervous system, which is always developing. Alcohol can affect a fetus at any time during the pregnancy.

Examples of teratogens include thalidomide, aminopterin, phenytoin, valproic acid, warfarin, ACE inhibitors, isotretinoin (Accutane), lithium, diazepam, phenothiazine, SSRIs, diethylstilbestrol, alcohol, tobacco, and androgens. Certain maternal infections can lead to birth defects in the fetus, such as chickenpox, hepatitis, AIDS, parvovirus, toxoplasmosis, Rubella, cytomegalovirus, herpes simplex virus, and syphilis (among others).

Key Takeaways

- Toxicology screening in the emergency department can be done on urine, saliva, or blood (but can rarely be assessed with other body fluids and hair).

- CNS toxicity can involve exposure to an agent that either excites the CNS or depresses the CNS.

- Cardiotoxicity or exposure to substances known to be toxic to the heart can involve problems with the heart rhythm, the heart muscle, or the blood pressure.

- Toxicity to the lungs by a toxin usually starts with pneumonitis, which is short-lived, but is followed by long-lasting fibrosis of the lungs.

- Toxicity related to the ear may be permanent or temporary, and may involve either hearing or the vestibular/balance system.

- Teratogens are toxic substances that may have an adverse effect on an embryo or fetus at any point in the gestation after about 10 days gestation.

Quiz

1. When evaluating a patient with a toxic exposure, you note that the patient has confusion, increased respirations, increased pulse, and increased blood pressure. What toxidrome does this represent?

a. Sympathomimetic toxidrome

b. Opioid toxidrome

c. Solvent toxidrome

d. Convulsant toxidrome

Answer: a. The sympathomimetic toxidrome involves symptoms, including confusion, increased respirations, increased pulse, and increased blood pressure. The toxin is likely a sympathomimetic drug or chemical.

2. In evaluating a patient who has a suspected toxic exposure, you note that the patient has irritation of skin exposed to the toxin, irritation of mucous membranes, and irritation of the GI tract. What toxidrome does this usually represent?

a. Sympathomimetic toxidrome

b. Opioid toxidrome

c. Solvent toxidrome

d. Corrosive toxidrome

Answer: d. This constellation of symptoms most fits with the corrosive toxidrome, which involves a toxic exposure with a corrosive agent.

3. The patient has admitted to an overdose of an opioid. What symptoms would you likely see?

a. CNS agitation

b. Seizures

c. Respiratory depression

d. Excessive sweating

Answer: c. In the opioid toxidrome, there is CNS depression, respiratory depression, and pinpoint pupils.

4. Which type of CNS response to a toxin will likely lead to rhabdomyolysis and kidney failure if not treated?

a. Psychomotor agitation

b. Delirium

c. Dementia

d. Brief seizure activity

Answer: a. Psychomotor agitation can cause myoglobin to be released from the muscle cells. The myoglobin can go to the kidneys and can cause kidney failure.

5. There are key similarities and differences between dementia and delirium. What are major differences between the two?

a. Delirium is slow-acting and dementia is fast-acting.

b. Delirium involves an altered state of consciousness and dementia does not.

c. Delirium involves an alteration in concentration and dementia does not.

d. Delirium is not treatable and dementia is treatable.

Answer: b. The main differences between delirium and dementia are that delirium is fluctuating in course and has an altered state of consciousness, while dementia does not have these features. Delirium comes on quickly and is treatable, while dementia is generally not treatable.

6. Delirium can be an effect from the taking of a drug or the withdrawal of a drug. Which scenario is least likely to result in delirium?

   a. Cocaine ingestion

   b. Amphetamine ingestion

   c. Benzodiazepine withdrawal

   d. Atropine withdrawal

Answer: d. The taking of atropine will cause delirium; however, the withdrawal from atropine won't likely cause delirium. The other scenarios will cause delirium, however.

7. For what purpose is flumazenil in treating toxic exposures or overdoses?

   a. For opiate overdoses

   b. For organophosphate exposures

   c. For hallucinogen exposures

   d. For benzodiazepine overdoses

Answer: d. Flumazenil is a specific antidote used it treating suspected benzodiazepine overdoses but it can precipitate seizures in patients who have been chronically taking benzodiazepines.

8. There are many drugs that can lead to renal toxicity. Which drug is least likely to cause renal toxicity?

   a. Acetaminophen

   b. Ibuprofen

   c. Gentamycin

   d. IV contrast dye

Answer: a. All of the above drugs are known for nephrotoxicity except for acetaminophen, which is known mainly for liver toxicity.

9. Certain chemotherapy drugs can cause lung toxicity. Which chemotherapy drug is not typically known for causing lung toxicity?

a. Bleomycin

b. Daunorubicin

c. Adarubicin

d. Arsenic trioxide

Answer: b. Daunorubicin isn't particularly known for causing lung toxicity; however, the others are known for this.

10. Which of the following drugs is not generally considered a teratogen?

a. Isotretinoin

b. Thalidomide

c. Phenytoin

d. Acetaminophen

Answer: d. All of the above choices are considered teratogens except for acetaminophen, which is not generally considered a teratogen and is safe to take in pregnancy.

Summary

This course was intended to discuss the numerous critical care issues and emergency management issues faced by the emergency medicine practitioner. The practice of emergency medicine involves the care of many different types of patients, some of whom are critically-ill, while others only have illnesses requiring observation and the basics of management. This course covered the basics of emergency medicine presentations as well as the emergency medicine workup techniques necessary to identify serious medical problems.

The first aspect in the care of the critically-ill, injured, or compromised patient is the establishment of an airway, which was the first topic covered in the first chapter of this course. The care of these individuals requires an evaluation of the individual's airway patency and the ability of the patient to take a spontaneous breath. For either problem, the patient will need an artificial airway. This first chapter was all about the evaluation and practice of airway management in the patient who requires oxygenation.

The second chapter of the course involved the phenomenon of "shock". The definition of shock is more complex that just the finding of low blood pressure. There are a wide variety of systemic complications that occur because of shock, the most serious of which is end-organ failure of the major organs, such as the kidneys and liver. This chapter covered two of the more common types of shock seen in emergency medicine, including cardiogenic shock and distributive shock.

Cardiac resuscitation was the topic of the third chapter of the course. Cardiac resuscitation is the emergency medical response to a cardiac arrest situation, which, in turn, usually results from a severe myocardial infarction with a severe arrhythmia, although things like a pulmonary embolism, ventricular wall rupture, low potassium levels, heavy exercise, and major blood loss can cause a cardiac arrest. This chapter discussed the pathophysiology of the cardiac arrest as well as the emergency medical response to this type of catastrophic event.

The topic of fever was covered in the fourth chapter of the course. One of the more common things an emergency medicine physician will have to deal with is the febrile patient. Most patients with fever will have some type of infection that needs to be discovered and managed. Less commonly, the cause of fever will be unrelated to an infection. This chapter focused on the typical febrile patient, including the workup of fever, the diagnosis of fever, and the treatment of fever and febrile illnesses.

Chest pain was the main topic of chapter five in this course. Chest pain in the adult emergency department patient can be serious or benign but always need to be worked up by the emergency room physician in order to identify which types of chest pain need further intervention and which can simply be monitored. This chapter discussed both the phenomenon of chest pain and the possible things that can cause this important symptom.

The sixth chapter in the course covered the emergency medicine topic of head trauma. The head trauma patient may have a concussion or other minor injury and they may have either an open head injury (penetrating) or a closed head injury (blunt trauma). Injuries can also be very severe, resulting in severe brain contusions and intracerebral bleeding that can be life-threatening if not treated quickly and aggressively.

The seventh chapter in the course involved a thorough discussion of eye injuries. Injury is the most common reason for eye-related emergency department visits. The incidence of eye injuries requiring emergency department medical attention in the US is estimated to be between 500 and 1000 patients per 100,000 population. This chapter covered some of the more common eye injuries seen in emergency medicine along with the treatment of these diseases.

The eighth chapter of the course involved the impact of chest trauma in an emergency department patient. Chest trauma can occur secondary to many different things, including penetrating injuries, falls, and motor vehicle accidents. The different things that can cause chest trauma can affect the heart or the lungs, leading to cardiorespiratory compromise. This chapter covered both blunt traumatic injuries of the chest and penetrating injuries of the chest.

The ninth chapter in the course included a discussion of abdominal trauma and its manifestations. Because there are many vital organs in the abdomen and pelvis, trauma to these areas is hardly ever benign. The patient with abdominal trauma can have damage to any of the solid organs in the abdomen or any part of the abdominal viscus. Infections tend to be common late manifestations of abdominal trauma as the viscus of the abdomen carries billions of microorganisms—some of them pathogenic. The purpose of this chapter was to discuss the basics of blunt abdominal trauma and its management.

The tenth chapter in this course was devoted to discussing the evaluation and management of the acute abdomen and the related phenomenon of pelvic pain. These are common problems in emergency medicine and require a systematic approach that attempts to distinguish between a non-operative condition and those that require surgical intervention. The definition of the "acute abdomen" is one that ultimately needs surgery to treat the patient's abdominal or pelvic complaints.

The major topic discussed in chapter eleven was the management of patients with multiple trauma. It is not uncommon for the emergency room physician to encounter a patient who has the confounding problem of having multiple areas of trauma secondary to a motor vehicle accident, a fall, or other serious injury. These patients need to be managed in a manner that addresses the more serious problems first, followed by a systematic assessment and management of the less serious injuries.

The emergency care of lacerations and other wounds was the primary topic of the twelfth chapter in the course. The treatment of skin wounds includes mainly the treatment of lacerations, abrasions, and puncture wounds—each of which are treated slightly differently. These are extremely common skin problems affecting nearly everyone at some point in their lives. The goal of the emergency medical physician or dermatologist is to determine what kind of wound the patient has and to use the proper protocols for each of these skin wounds. The focus of this chapter was on the management of wounds and the specific techniques used in emergency laceration repair.

Chapter thirteen of the course involved the care and management of psychiatric emergencies. A psychiatric emergency can be defined as any situation in which the healthcare provider confronts a situation in which the patient cannot stop acting on compulsions to harm themselves or another person. The patient may present with full awareness of the impact of their desired behavior but more often than not, they present with a lack of judgment and insight into what might happen should they follow through on their compulsion.

The study of toxicology in the emergency department was the topic of the fourteenth chapter of the book. This involved both the study of toxic medications that are not normally toxic under typical situations but become toxic in high doses and a discussion of things that are always toxic to the body. There are some things that are toxic to the kidneys, toxic to the heart, toxic to the lungs, toxic to a growing fetus, or toxic to the ears. Each of these was discussed in this chapter.

Course Questions and Answers

1. For what reason should the airflow rate be low in bag-valve mask ventilations?

   a. To avoid alveolar trauma

   b. To avoid gastric inflation with air

   c. To avoid a pneumothorax

   d. To avoid airway distention

Answer: b. The main reason why a low airflow rate is used in bag-valve mask ventilations is to reduce gastric inflation with air.

2. Why should the mask in a bag-valve mask be as small as possible?

   a. There is less dead space with a small mask.

   b. This type of mask works best for people with facial hair.

   c. it prevents coverage of the nose and only covers the mouth.

   d. it can be used in a single-person procedure but not a two-person procedure.

Answer: a. A small mask in a BMV device will provide for a decreased dead space and better ventilations.

3. About what is the average size of an ETT used in an adult patient?

   a. 5 mm

   b. 6 mm

   c. 7 mm

   d. 8 mm

Answer: c. The average size of an ET tube in adults is about 7 mm internal diameter.

4. What is the major indication for a surgical airway versus intubation?

   a. Epiglottis

   b. Massive facial and airway trauma

   c. Cervical spine injury

   d. Need for prolonged ventilation

Answer: b. Patients with massive facial and airway trauma have the highest need for a surgical airway as intubation can be technically difficult.

5. In evaluating the patient needing a possible intubation, what aspect of the "LEMON" mnemonic cannot be done in a patient with a suspected cervical spinal cord injury?

a. N

b. O

c. M

d. E

Answer: a. The "N" part of the mnemonic refers to neck mobility, which cannot be assessed when the patient is in a cervical collar is suspected of having a cervical spinal cord injury.

6. In a rapid sequence induction, which drug would be given first?

a. Succinylcholine

b. Propofol

c. Acetylcholine

d. Vecuronium

Answer: b. Propofol is the first step in the RSI procedure as it creates an unconscious state.

7. You have placed an ET tube and want to know if it is placed properly. What is the best way to make sure the ETT placement has been successful?

a. PA chest x-ray

b. AP chest x-ray

c. End-tidal CO_2 measurement

d. Lung auscultation

Answer: c. The best way to know if the ET tube is in correct placement is to do an end-tidal CO_2 level measurement, which will tell if ventilation is adequate. The other tests can be done but are not as accurate as the end-tidal CO_2 measurement.

8. In which patient would the LMA device be preferred over ETT placement?

a. Trauma patient with cervical spine injury

b. Septic patient who is semi-conscious

c. Cardiac arrest patient in the field

d. Tension pneumothorax patient

Answer: a. A trauma patient with a suspected cervical spine injury might do better with an LMA device as it doesn't require tipping of the neck to visualize the vocal cords.

9. In inserting the LMA, what is the first step necessary to do this intubation?

a. Place the patient in a sniffing position

b. Inflate the cuff to inspect it for leaks

c. Lubricate the tube and cuff

d. Give etomidate to render the patient unconscious

Answer: b. The first step in inserting the LMA is to inflate the cuff and inspect it for leaks before deflating it again and preparing it for the intubation.

10. In performing a surgical airway, where is the entry point of the airway?

a. Thyroid cartilage

b. Between the first and second ring of the trachea

c. Cricothyroid membrane

d. Hypopharynx

Answer: c. The surgical airway is performed so that the entry point of the airway is the cricothyroid membrane.

11. What size tracheostomy tube should be placed through the cricothyroid membrane when the surgical airway procedure is being performed?

a. 4.0

b. 5.0

c. 6.0

d. 7.0

Answer: a. A 4.0-sized tracheostomy tube is the right-sized tube for an adult patient having a cricothyroidotomy.

12. When can the Swans-Ganz catheter be used in a therapeutic setting?

a. Pulmonary hypertension treatment

b. Aspiration of air embolism in the pulmonary vasculature

c. To assist in a coronary angioplasty

d. To remove a pulmonary embolism

Answer: b. A therapeutic reason for having a Swans-Ganz catheter in place is to aspirate an air embolism in the pulmonary vasculature.

13. In which setting should the Swan-Ganz catheter probably not be use?

a. Symptomatic valvular disease

b. Acute heart failure

c. Sepsis or septicemia

d. Severe CAD

Answer: a. This type of catheter should not be used in cases of symptomatic valvular disease, especially with aortic and mitral valve disease or in cases of a prosthetic valve problem.

14. Where should be the site of insertion of the PAC be when hemorrhaging is expected?

    a. Right subclavian vein

    b. Left subclavian vein

    c. Right jugular vein

    d. Left femoral vein

Answer: d. The left or right femoral vein insertion is more technically difficult, when it comes to the insertion of the PAC but is preferable when hemorrhaging is suspected.

15. What is the maximum recommended dose of dopamine in cases of cardiogenic shock?

    a. 5 mcg/kg/min

    b. 10 mcg/kg/min

    c. 15 mcg/kg/min

    d. 20 mcg/kg/min

Answer: d. The maximum recommended dose of dopamine is 20 mcg/kg/min.

16. What might the advantage be of using dobutamine in cases of cardiogenic shock over dopamine?

    a. It raises the MAP faster than dopamine

    b. It causes a lesser myocardial oxygen demand.

    c. It increases the renal vascular perfusion to a greater degree.

    d. Much larger doses can be incorporated as part of the treatment.

Answer: b. It can be better than dopamine because it causes a lesser myocardial oxygen demand.

17. In the definitive management for cardiogenic shock, what is the treatment of choice?

    a. Thrombolytic therapy

    b. Heparin therapy

    c. Percutaneous coronary angioplasty

    d. Dobutamine therapy

Answer: c. The definitive treatment of choice is a PCI or percutaneous coronary angioplasty, which can restore blood flow to the coronary arterial system. If this is not possible, a CABG procedure should be done. A second-line therapy is thrombolytic therapy.

18. What is the most common cause of distributive shock?

a. Addisonian crisis

b. Toxic shock syndrome

c. Sepsis

d. Anaphylaxis

Answer: c. Sepsis is the leading cause of distributive shock, even though the other choices can cause this type of shock as well.

19. What is the underlying pathophysiology behind distributive shock?

    a. Systemic vasodilation of the arteries.

    b. Decreased cardiac output.

    c. Volume depletion.

    d. Decreased cardiac preload

Answer: a. The main pathophysiological issue behind distributive shock is systemic vasodilation.

20. Which type of shock is most associated with a traumatic injury?

    a. Distributive shock

    b. Hypovolemic shock

    c. Cardiogenic shock

    d. Obstructive shock

Answer: b. Trauma is most commonly linked to hypovolemic shock, which is best treated with volume replacement.

21. The diagnosis of SIRS (systemic inflammatory response syndrome) is based on several criteria. Which is not included in the criteria?

    a. Abnormalities in WBC

    b. Abnormalities in heart rate

    c. Abnormalities in temperature

    d. Abnormalities in hematocrit

Answer: d. All of the above are criteria used to identify patients with SIRS except for the hematocrit, which is not a part of this disorder.

22. About what percentage of septic patients with distributive shock will have disseminated intravascular coagulation?

    a. Five percent

    b. Twenty percent

c. Fifty percent

d. Eighty percent

Answer: c. About fifty percent of patients will have some degree of disseminated intravascular coagulation or DIC.

23. The patient suffered an out-of-hospital cardiac arrest from a non-cardiac condition. What is the most common cause of a non-cardiac cardiac arrest?

    a. Trauma

    b. Internal bleeding

    c. Drug overdose

    d. Drowning

Answer: a. Trauma is the most common cause of a cardiac arrest not secondary to a heart problem. The other choices are much less likely to cause this.

24. What is the gold standard in determining the presence of a cardiac arrest?

    a. Apnea

    b. Lack of carotid pulse

    c. Unconsciousness

    d. Lack of movement

Answer: b. The gold standard for determining the presence of a cardiac arrest is a lack of a carotid pulse. The other findings are not considered the gold standard in clinically diagnosing a cardiac arrest.

25. In a BLS situation, what is considered the most effect component of this protocol?

    a. Artificial respirations

    b. Sweeping the mouth

    c. Heimlich maneuver

    d. Chest compressions

Answer: d. Chest compressions are considered the most effective component of the BLS protocol.

26. The patient has had a cardiac arrest and Is found to have systole. What is the approximate length of time that CPR should be given before stopping?

    a. 10 minutes

    b. 20 minutes

    c. 30 minutes

    d. 69 minutes

Answer: b. In asystole, the patient should have CPR performed for approximately 20 minutes before stopping.

27. In which clinical situation should the period of CPR be extended in an out-of-hospital cardiac arrest?

    a. Infant with asystole in an unwitnessed arrest

    b. Middle-aged alcoholic with known CAD

    c. Young adult who is hypothermic when found

    d. Pregnant female with asystole secondary to trauma

Answer: c. In the young adult who is hypothermic when found, CPR should continue until the patient is warmed.

28. Which drug is least likely to be recommended in a cardiac arrest situation?

    a. Amiodarone

    b. Calcium

    c. Atropine

    d. Vasopressin

Answer: b. Calcium is generally not warranted in a cardiac arrest situation and may make things worse. The same is true of bicarbonate administration.

29. The use of atropine is used in what clinical situation in a cardiac arrest?

    a. Asystole

    b. Pulseless electrical activity

    c. Bradycardia

    d. Supraventricular tachycardia

Answer: c. Atropine is only indicated in cases of bradycardia and is no longer recommended in asystole or pulseless electrical activity

30. Under what situation should therapeutic thermoregulation be employed?

    a. Near drowning

    b. Unconsciousness after resuscitation

    c. Hypothermic patient after resuscitation

    d. Febrile child after resuscitation

Answer: b. The main advantage of therapeutic thermoregulation is to lower the body temperature after return of a pulse in patient who is still unconscious. It is done for 24 hours and has been found to improve survival and lessen disability.

31. What is the range of temperature aimed for during therapeutic thermoregulation?

    a. 85-90 degrees

    b. 90-97 degrees

    c. 95-98 degrees

    d. 99-101 degrees

Answer: b. Patients requiring therapeutic thermoregulation are cooled to a range of temperatures between 90 and 97 degrees for 24 hours after resuscitation.

32. The lack of what feature in resuscitation improves the survival rate?

    a. Recognizing a pre-arrest situation

    b. Early intubation

    c. Urgent CPR when the patient is in a cardiac arrest situation

    d. Revascularization procedure soon after resuscitation

Answer: b. All of the above are chain of survival events that improve the outcome of the patient except for early intubation, which will not necessarily improve survival.

33. Under what circumstances should a precordial thump be entertained?

    a. In a patient with a witnessed, monitored arrest.

    b. In any type of witnessed arrest.

    c. When asystole has been found on the monitor strip.

    d. In a young person with any type of arrest.

Answer: a. The precordial thump should be used in any witnessed, monitored arrest when VTach has been found without a pulse.

34. The goal with a cardiac arrest is to be discharged with normal mentation. What percentage of arrest patients who are discharged from the hospital have normal CNS statuses?

    a. 2 percent

    b. 34 percent

    c. 65 percent

    d. 89 percent

Answer: d. In those who survive their out of hospital arrest, about 89 percent will be discharge with a normal CNS status.

35. In the febrile child with vomiting or fever, which would be the least acceptable choice for rehydration?

    a. Water

    b. Sports drinks

    c. Gelatin

    d. Soup

Answer: b. Sports drinks contain a great deal of sugar, which tends to make diarrhea worse and will worsen the dehydration. The other rehydration sources are considered good ways to hydrate a febrile child.

36. A fever in an elderly patient can be identified in any of the following ways. Which definition does not fit the criteria for a fever in an elderly adult?

    a. An axillary temperature reading of at least 98 degrees Fahrenheit.

    b. An oral temperature reading of at least 100 degrees Fahrenheit.

    c. Two oral temperature readings of at least 99 degrees Fahrenheit.

    d. An increase in body temperature of more than 2 degrees over the baseline body temperature.

Answer: a. Axillary temperatures are notoriously poor ways to measure the temperature in an elderly adult so this should not be the basis for a fever. The other choices represent fever in an elderly person.

37. In evaluating a febrile elderly person, what is the first test that should be performed as part of the evaluation?

    a. Urinalysis

    b. Urine culture

    c. CBC with differential

    d. Chest x-ray

Answer: c. The initial test of a CBC with differential will be able to tell the difference between a likely bacterial infection and a non-bacterial source of a fever so this is a good test to perform.

38. When should a skin biopsy and culture most likely be obtained in a suspected skin infection?

    a. When the patient is diabetic.

    b. When the skin shows moist ulcerations.

    c. When there are bullous lesions of the skin.

d. When the initial antimicrobial choice fails to work.

Answer: d. In general, the only appropriate time to get a skin culture is if the initial antimicrobial therapy fails to be effective in treating the problem.

39. You suspect that a diabetic patient with an ankle ulcer has osteomyelitis as a cause of their fever. What can you do first to evaluate the patient as possibly having this problem?

    a. Bone biopsy

    b. MRI of the ankle

    c. CT scan of the ankle

    d. Plain x-ray of the ankle

Answer: b. The best test and the most sensitive test for osteomyelitis in this situation would be an MRI of the bone, which will lead to a bone biopsy for organisms if this test is positive for a bone infection.

40. The patient is suspected of having a mucocutaneous fungal infection of the skin. What is the initial test of choice?

    a. Fungal cultures of the skin surface

    b. Skin biopsy looking for fungal pathogens

    c. KOH smear of a tissue scraping

    d. No testing is recommended

Answer: c. If a fungal infection of the skin is suspected, a KOH smear of a tissue scraping should be obtained, which can quickly confirm the presence of yeast or dermatophytes.

41. The patient has bloody diarrhea, fever, and abdominal cramping. You obtain a stool culture and identify an organism. Which would be the least likely organism to isolate in this type of culture?

    a. Giardia

    b. Campylobacter

    c. Shigella

    d. Salmonella

Answer: a. Giardia is a protozoal species that will likely yield watery diarrhea. It will also not be able to be cultured in a typical stool culture. The other species would be identifiable in a stool culture.

42. You are caring for an older patient with severe abdominal pain, fever, and ileus. What test will least likely help identify the source of the infection?

    a. CT scan of the abdomen

    b. Ultrasound of the abdomen

    c. Upper GI endoscopy

d. MRI scan of the abdomen

Answer: c. This patient has some sort of intraabdominal infection but is unlikely to show organisms or pathology in an upper GI endoscopy. An imaging study of the abdomen will show the presence of an abscess or other focus of infection.

43. A fever in a child lasting how long should be evaluated if the child is under the age of two years?

    a. One day

    b. Two days

    c. Three days

    d. Seven days

Answer: a. Any fever lasting twenty-four hours or longer in a child under the age of two years should be evaluated in the emergency room or clinic.

44. You believe a patient with a fever has an infectious disease because of a rash. Which infectious disease are you least likely to associate with the finding of a rash?

    a. Rocky Mountain spotted fever

    b. Scarlet fever

    c. Rheumatic fever

    d. Acute otitis media

Answer: d. All of the above are infectious diseases that will cause rashes except for acute otitis media, which rarely yields a rash.

45. Which ECG finding is least predictive of an acute MI as a cause of chest pain in the emergency patient?

    a. ST segment elevation

    b. Hyperacute T waves

    c. Short PR interval

    d. New onset left bundle branch block

Answer: c. All of the above are considered suspicious for an acute MI except for a short PR interval, which is not predictive of an acute MI.

46. You are evaluating the possibility of a patient having an acute MI who has an equivocal ECG reading. Which clinical finding least likely portends the presence of an acute MI?

    a. Pressure-like chest pain

    b. Pain radiating tot the neck, back, shoulders, jaw, or arm

    c. Male older than 60 years of age

d. Slender build

Answer: d. The findings noted above portend the presence of an acute MI except for slender build, which points away from an MI.

47. What is the most common musculoskeletal chest pain diagnosis seen in children?

    a. Precordial catch

    b. Fractured rib

    c. Costochondritis

    d. Lower rib pain syndrome

Answer: a. In children and young people, the most common musculoskeletal chest pain diagnosis is the precordial catch.

48. Why are risk scores important in identifying ACS patients?

    a. Because they better predict death and MI than just one test.

    b. Because ST segment elevation alone doesn't predict MI in all cases as the ECG may be normal.

    c. Because it avoids treating people unnecessarily who are low risk.

    d. For all of the above reasons.

Answer: d. Risk scores help identify high risk populations, are better predictors of mortality, help identify patients who don't have typical ST-segment elevation, and avoids treating low-risk patients unnecessarily.

49. What is not considered a preliminary treatment in the care of a patient with chest pain secondary to a NSTEMI infarction?

    a. Clopidogrel

    b. Revascularization

    c. Heparin

    d. Aspirin

Answer: b. The initial agents that are given for NSTEMI infarction include clopidogrel, heparin, aspirin, fentanyl, and nitroglycerin, with revascularization procedures representing later definitive treatment when possible.

50. Which patient is a good candidate for nitrate therapy as they have no major contraindications for their use?

    a. The hypertensive patient

    b. The patient with a right ventricular infarction

    c. The patient with a pericardial effusion

d. The patient with recent phosphodiesterase-5 inhibitor therapy

Answer: a. All of the above patients have contraindications to nitrate therapy with the exception of the hypertensive patient, who is a good candidate for nitrate therapy.

51. Beta-blocker therapy is indicated in most cases of ACS. Which drug is the treatment of choice for this?

    a. Metoprolol

    b. Labetalol

    c. Propranolol

    d Nadolol

Answer: a. The best and most often-used treatment for ACS when it comes to beta-blocker therapy is metoprolol, given IV every five minutes for a maximal dose of 15 mg IV, followed by oral therapy.

52. Why is clopidogrel often withheld from the suspected ACS patient until after they have an angiogram?

    a. Because it causes excess bleeding in angiography procedures.

    b. Because it doesn't affect mortality unless the patient has advanced three-vessel disease.

    c. Because it must be withheld in patients who need a CABG procedure.

    d. Because it only reduces mortality if it is given late in the evaluation of the disease process.

Answer: c. It is often withheld until after the angiogram because patients found to need a CABG need to have the clopidogrel withheld until after the bypass procedure.

53. What is the major side effect/risk factor in giving a patient clopidogrel in acute coronary syndrome?

    a. Intracerebral hemorrhage

    b. Upper GI bleeding

    c. Lower GI bleeding

    d. Nosebleeds

Answer: b. The most common risk of giving a patient clopidogrel therapy is that they may have upper GI bleeding.

54. You are caring for a high-risk patient who you plan to give clopidogrel therapy to. What can you give them to reduce their risk of complications?

    a. Prednisone

    b. Histamine-2 blocker therapy

    c. Antacid therapy

d. Omeprazole therapy

Answer: d. Omeprazole is a PPI that will reduce the risk of clopidogrel therapy complications, which is mainly upper GI bleeding.

55. In patients with chest pain and evidence of unstable angina or NSTEMI, what would be the definitive treatment of choice if at all possible?

    a. Revascularization with a PCI

    b. Aspirin and clopidogrel therapy

    c. Tissue plasminogen activator therapy

    d. Morphine and nitroglycerin therapy

Answer: a. While all of the above choices are possible, the treatment that will definitively help these patients is a percutaneous coronary intervention procedure with the goal being revascularization. The other treatment options are not definitive therapies.

56. What is the main complication of a subdural hematoma?

    a. Skull fracture

    b. Increased intracranial pressure

    c. Cervical spine injury

    d. Anemia from blood loss

Answer: b. The main complication of a subdural hematoma is increased intracranial pressure, which can damage the brain tissue.

57. Which type of intracranial bleed has the worsened short-term prognosis?

    a. Chronic subdural hematoma

    b. Acute subdural hematoma

    c. Subarachnoid hemorrhage

    d. Epidural hematoma

Answer: b. An epidural hematoma involves brisk arterial bleeding that results in acute death if not aggressively managed, but the rate of death is higher in acute subdural hematomas.

58. What is the approximate mortality rate from patients with an acute subdural hematoma?

    a. 40 percent

    b. 60 percent

    c. 80 percent

    d. 95 percent

Answer: c. The rate of death from an acute subdural hematoma is about 80 percent.

59. What criterion is not listed as a defining factor in a mild traumatic brain injury?

    a. Seizure activity

    b. Brief loss of consciousness

    c. Negative CT scan findings

    d. Amnesia for the event

Answer: a. The presence of seizure activity is more common in severe TBI and is rarely seen in mild TBI.

60. About how long should a patient be in a vegetative state in order to have the diagnosis of persistent vegetative state?

    a. One week

    b. One month

    c. Three months

    d. Six months

Answer: b. A persistent vegetative state involves being in a vegetative state for a minimum of one month.

61. What is the diagnostic imaging of choice in identifying cases of traumatic brain injury?

    a. Ultrasound of the brain

    b. MRI of the brain

    c. SPECT scan of the brain

    d. CT scan without contrast

Answer: d. A CT scan without contrast will show abnormalities of the brain and bleeding within the skull, making it the diagnostic imaging of choice in identifying TBI in most people.

62. What is the most diffuse injury that can happen to the brain in a traumatic brain injury?

    a. Diffuse axonal injury

    b. Contracoup injury

    c. Subdural hematoma

    d. Penetrating injury to the brain

Answer: a. The diffuse axonal injury involves widespread areas of white matter damage involving wide areas of the brain. This is the most diffuse injury that can happen to the brain in a traumatic brain injury.

63. In what type of traumatic brain injury is the MRI scan preferable as a diagnostic tool over any other modality?

    a. Basilar skull fracture

    b. Subarachnoid hemorrhage

    c. Diffuse axonal injury

    d. Contrecoup injury

Answer: c. The only time that MRI scanning is preferable to CT scanning when diffuse axonal injury is suspected.

64. Which is considered the most severe complication of a head injury?

    a. Brainstem herniation

    b. Seizure disorder

    c. Prolonged coma

    d. Focal neurological deficit

Answer: a. The brainstem herniation is considered the most severe type of complication of a head injury, likely leading to respiratory distress and death.

65. Which athlete is most likely to have chronic traumatic encephalopathy?

    a. Soccer player

    b. Football player

    c. Track and field athlete

    d. Swimmer

Answer: b. Chronic traumatic encephalopathy or CTE occurs mainly in athletes who sustain multiple head injuries. It is found mainly in football players and boxers.

66. What is not considered a standard treatment in the care of the patient with a severe TBI?

    a. Sedation

    b. Elevation of the head of the bed

    c. Anticonvulsant therapy

    c. ICP monitoring

Answer: c. All of the above are indicated in treating the severe TBI patient except for anticonvulsant therapy, which is rarely necessary in the acute phase of treatment.

67. What is not a recommended part of the management of a corneal abrasion?

    a. Visual inspection for a foreign body

b. Fluorescein staining of the eye under the microscope

c. Patching the affected eye

d. Removing possible rust rings

Answer: c. All of the above are recommended treatments for a corneal foreign body except for the patching of the eye, which is not recommended as it increases the risk of secondary infection.

68. You are instructing the patient who got a fish hook in his eye that is still there. What should you give him as far as advice?

a. Remove the fish hook as soon as possible.

b. Follow up within 24 hours to an ophthalmologist.

c. Flush the eye with water until all debris is removed.

d. Cover the eye with a paper cup and present to the emergency department.

Answer: d. The only acceptable recommendation is to cover the eye and present immediately without flushing the eye out or removing the foreign body.

69. What is the more harmful chemical for a person to get into the eye?

a. Sodium hydroxide

b. Hydrochloric acid

c. Acetic acid

d. Nail polish remover

Answer: a. Sodium hydroxide is an alkaline substance that is most likely to cause a permanent change in the appearance of the eye and in its ability to later have normal vision.

70. What is not considered a good treatment for a hyphema?

a. Beta-blocker therapy

b. Atropine eye drops

c. Antibiotic eye drops

d. Avoidance of blood thinners

Answer: c. All of the above treatments are useful for the treatment of a hyphema with the exception of antibiotic eye drops, which are not necessary as this is a bleeding problem.

71. What is the definitive treatment for a blowout fracture of the eye?

a. Patching the eye for up to two weeks

b. Ice application to the eye for 48 hours

c. Flushing the eye to remove debris from the fracture

d. Surgical intervention to remove trapped muscles within the fracture site.

Answer: d. The definitive treatment for a blowout fracture is to remove the trapped muscles surgically as there is no effective medical or first-aid treatment for this problem.

72. The patient has the complaint of sudden vision loss over 12 hours. What is least likely to cause this problem?

   a. Vitreous opacification

   b. Ocular contusion

   c. Retinal detachment

   d. Optic nerve infarction

Answer: b. Any of the above can cause sudden vision loss except for an ocular contusion, which will generally not affect the vision.

73. Which causes of loss of vision will not have cardiac risk factors as a past medical history?

   a. Transient ischemic attack

   b. Retinal artery occlusion

   c. Amaurosis fugax

   d. Ocular migraine

Answer: d. An ocular migraine will have vision loss but will not have cardiac risk factors as a part of their past medical history.

74. Which vision loss cause can best be diagnosed with gonioscopy.

   a. Acute narrow-angle glaucoma

   b. Endophthalmitis

   c. Corneal ulcer

   d. Retinal detachment

Answer: a. Patients with acute narrow-angle glaucoma can be diagnosed with a gonioscopy evaluation that would show elevations of the intraocular pressure.

75. Which type of vision loss is least likely to be determined by the finding of an abnormal fundoscopy evaluation?

   a. Retinal detachment

   b. Cerebrovascular accident

   c. Central retinal artery occlusion

   d. Central retinal vein occlusion

Answer: b. All of the above have specific findings on a fundoscopy evaluation except for a CVA, which will have normal findings on a fundoscopy evaluation.

76. The patient is being evaluated for a unilateral vision loss on the right side. They have an absence of a direct pupillary reflex on the right but a normal consensual response. What does this suggest?

    a. Ocular migraine

    b. Central retinal artery occlusion

    c. Optic nerve damage

    d. Corneal ulcer

Answer: c. This set of findings most suggests an optic nerve issue as the consensual reflex is normal.

77. What finding would most likely lead to vision loss secondary to a corneal ulcer?

    a. Recent eye trauma

    b. Cerebrovascular disease

    c. Recent eye surgery

    d. Excessive contact use

Answer: d. The excessive use of contact lenses can lead to a corneal ulcer and unilateral or bilateral vision loss.

78. What is not considered an urgent reason for doing heart or great vessel surgery after blunt trauma?

    a. Radiographic evidence of great vessel injury

    b. Cardiac tamponade

    c. Pulmonary embolism

    d. Aortic aneurysm

Answer: d. There is no evidence to suggest that an aortic aneurysm is new so if there is no active bleeding the injury can be treated with a laser surgery.

79. What is the most common injury sustained in a blunt chest trauma injury?

    a. Cardiac contusion

    b. Rib fracture

    c. Sternal fracture

    d. Hemothorax

Answer: b. The rib fracture is the most common injury seen in blunt chest trauma. The other choices are much less common.

80. What is not considered a mainstay of treatment for the pain of rib fractures?

    a. Oral NSAID therapy

    b. Intercostal nerve block

    c. Epidural anesthesia

    d. Surgical repair

Answer: d. All of the above can be used for rib fracture patients except for surgical repair, which is rarely recommended.

81. What is not considered one of the major underlying injuries associated with a sternal fracture?

    a. Rib fractures

    b. Subclavian arterial disruption

    c. Closed head injury

    d. Cardiac contusion

Answer: b. A subclavian artery disruption will be highly unlikely with a sternal fracture; however, the other findings can be seen with this type of fracture.

82. What is the main finding least likely to be seen in traumatic asphyxia?

    a. Petechiae of the face

    b. Scalp laceration

    c. Subconjunctival hemorrhages

    d. Periorbital bruising

Answer: b. All of the above are associated with traumatic asphyxia, except for scalp lacerations.

83. What is considered the main cause of the pneumothorax in blunt chest trauma?

    a. Barotrauma to the lungs

    b. Direct blow to the lungs

    c. Deceleration injury

    d. Rib fracture penetrating the lung

Answer: d. The main finding is that of a rib fracture that penetrates the lung, causing a pneumothorax.

84. Which blunt traumatic injury to the chest is associated with the highest mortality rate?

    a. Clavicle fracture

b. Bronchial disruption

c. Tension pneumothorax

d. Pulmonary contusion

Answer: b. The patient with a bronchial disruption has a high mortality rate with many patients not surviving to definitive treatment in the emergency department.

85. What is the treatment of choice for cardiac tamponade from blunt cardiac trauma?

    a. Surgical repair of the bleeding vessels

    b. Chest tube placement

    c. Pericardiocentesis

    d. No treatment necessary in most cases

Answer: c. The treatment of choice for cardiac tamponade is to perform an emergency pericardiocentesis in the emergency department, followed by definitive surgery if indicated.

86. What is the major pathophysiology behind an aortic injury and chest trauma?

    a. Deceleration injury

    b. Compression of the vessel by a blunt force

    c. Internal laceration of the aorta

    d. Contusion of the aorta leading to secondary aortic wall rupture

Answer: a. It is a deceleration injury that is most likely the underlying factor in aortic blunt chest injury.

87. What type of penetrating injury is considered the highest velocity injury to have?

    a. Handgun

    b. Shotgun

    c. Knife wound

    d. Blast injury

Answer: d. Blast injuries are the highest velocity injuries to have and are usually found in military-type injuries.

88. You evaluate a patient who has crepitus of the right lower anterior rib cage. What type of abdominal injury would you most likely suspect?

    a. Hepatic disruption

    b. Pancreatic laceration

    c. Diaphragmatic hernia

d. Splenic rupture

Answer: a. The finding of crepitus in the right lower rib cage most likely points to a hepatic injury, such as a rupture of the capsule or a hepatic laceration.

89. What imaging technique can be performed on a patient who is not hemodynamically stable but is suspected of having blunt abdominal trauma with hemoperitoneum?

    a. CT scan of the abdomen

    b. MRI of the abdomen

    c. FAST evaluation of the abdomen

    d. Flat and upright x-ray of the abdomen

Answer: c. The FAST evaluation is quick and portable. It is very sensitive for finding areas of bleeding within the blunt-traumatized abdomen.

90. Which is not considered one of the ultrasound windows obtained in a FAST examination?

    a. Peri-renal

    b. Peri-cardiac

    c. Peri-splenic

    d. Peri-hepatic

Answer: a. All of the above (plus the pelvic window) will be looked at in a FAST examination except for the peri-renal window, which does not exist as part of the examination.

91. Which organ or body area in the abdomen is most likely to be injured in blunt abdominal trauma?

    a. Liver

    b. Spleen

    c. Small intestines

    d. Pancreas

Answer: a. The liver is the most commonly organ involved in blunt abdominal traumatic injuries.

92. Which is not considered an indication for doing a laparotomy in a blunt trauma patient?

    a. Negative FAST evaluation

    b. Hypovolemic shock

    c. Peritonitis

    d. Clinical deterioration during the evaluation

Answer: a. Any of the above are signs indicating the need for laparotomy except for a negative FAST examination, which would be a reason not to do a laparotomy.

93. Which patients can easily be treated using nonoperative means?

    a. The patient with a ruptured small intestine

    b. The patient with a traumatic diaphragmatic hernia

    c. The pediatric patient with a hepatic laceration

    d. The patient with a fever and a rigid abdomen

Answer: c. Patients with a hepatic laceration, particularly the pediatric patient, can be treated using nonoperative means. The other patients will likely need a laparotomy.

94. How much IV fluid is the maximum amount that should be given before blood products are entertained?

    a. 500 ml

    b. 1000 ml

    c. 2000 ml

    d. 3000 ml

Answer: c. A total of 2 liters or 2000 ml IV crystalloid solution should be given before considering blood products instead.

95. What is the first x-ray that needs to be obtained in a patient suspected of having blunt abdominal trauma?

    a. FAST examination

    b. Supine chest x-ray

    c. Flat and upright of the abdomen

    d. CT scan of the abdomen

Answer: b. The first x-rays should be the supine chest x-ray, lateral cervical spine x-ray, and the pelvic x-ray. The FAST examination can be done after these tests have been performed.

96. In cases where the FAST examination is equivocal or negative but clinically, the patient still appears unstable, what is the next step?

    a. Perform a DPL procedure

    b. Get an MRI of the abdomen

    c. Get a CT scan of the abdomen

    d. Go directly to laparotomy

Answer: a. As the FAST examination may miss intra-abdominal bleeding, a DPL procedure can be done to check for bleeding within the abdomen. This is a fast procedure that can be done on patients who are mild to moderately hemodynamically unstable.

97. Which type of injury is most responsive to using arterial embolization in order to control hemorrhage?

a. Hepatic lacerations

b. Splenic lacerations

c. Ruptured small intestine

d. Renal capsular rupture

Answer: b. Patients with splenic lacerations can be treated nonoperatively using arterial embolization of the splenic artery, often with good success.

98. What is the most important factor driving the evaluation of the abdominal pain in suspected acute abdomen cases?

a. The location of the pain

b. The presence or absence of a fever

c. The severity of the pain

d. The presence or absence of nausea and vomiting

Answer: a. The location of the pain should drive the further evaluation of the pain in the emergency department.

99. Which type of pain is most likely to have a cardiac origin in the differential diagnosis?

a. Right upper quadrant pain

b. Left upper quadrant pain

c. Epigastric pain

d. Periumbilical pain

Answer: c. Epigastric pain may actually be secondary to a cardiac origin, such as a myocardial infarction.

100. Early appendicitis should be in the differential diagnosis of pain in what area?

a. Epigastrium

b. Periumbilical area

c. Left lower quadrant

d. Right upper quadrant

Answer: b. Pain in the periumbilical area is where early appendicitis usually presents itself so this should be in the differential diagnosis of this area of pain.

101.   You suspect a patient of hypovolemia secondary to acute GI bleeding. What test, besides a standard blood pressure can suggest this possibility?

a. Hematocrit

b. FAST examination

c. Orthostatic blood pressure readings

d. Upper GI endoscopy

Answer: c. Orthostatic blood pressure readings will document the hypovolemia. A FAST examination only works for traumatic sources of bleeding and an upper GI endoscopy will not help identify lower GI bleeding. A hematocrit will often be normal in the acute stages of GI bleeding.

102.   Which positive sign is most predictive of an abdominal wall pain as being the source of the patient's complaint?

a. Murphy's sign

b. Carnett's sign

c. Psoas sign

d. Cullen's sign

Answer: b. A positive Carnett's sign highly points to the abdominal wall as being the source of the patient's pain.

103.   Which positive sign is most predictive of pain being secondary to acute cholecystitis?

a. Murphy's sign

b. Carnett's sign

c. Psoas sign

d. Cullen's sign

Answer: a. A positive Murphy's sign is seen in 65 percent of cases of acute cholecystitis and moderately predicts this as the cause of the patient's pain.

104.   What type of gastrointestinal abnormality is best seen on a flat plate of the abdomen?

a. Acute cholelithiasis

b. Appendicitis

c. Paralytic ileus

d. Diverticulosis

Answer: c. A paralytic ileus can be demonstrated on a flat plate as it will show up with multiple dilated loops of bowel and air-fluid levels in the colon.

105. You suspect that a patient has an ectopic pregnancy. What type of imaging study would you most likely entertain?

a. Transabdominal ultrasound of the pelvis

b. CT scan of the pelvis

c. MRI of the pelvis

d. Transvaginal ultrasound of the pelvis

Answer: d. The diagnostic imaging study of choice in this situation would be a transvaginal ultrasound, which is 95 percent sensitive in detecting an ectopic pregnancy.

106. What laboratory testing in pregnant woman make the diagnosis of an acute abdomen more equivocal and difficult to make?

a. Renal function studies

b. WBC with differential

c. Liver function studies

d. Hemoglobin/hematocrit

Answer: b. Pregnant woman have a naturally-elevated WBC count, especially later in the pregnancy, making this a difficult test to interpret when an acute infection of the abdomen is suspected.

107. The patient you are evaluating is 34 weeks' gestation and has right upper quadrant abdominal pain. What is the least likely diagnosis in this case?

a. Acute cholecystitis

b. Peptic ulcer disease

c. HELLP syndrome

d. Hepatitis

Answer: b. All of the above choices would yield acute right upper quadrant abdominal pain except for peptic ulcer disease, which would lead to epigastric or left upper quadrant abdominal pain.

108. What medical specialist is the most important to have available when the multiply-injured patient is seen and managed in a tertiary care center?

a. Neurosurgery

b. Orthopedics

c. Cardiology

d. Gastroenterology

Answer: a. It is most important to have a neurosurgery specialist available with a multiply-injured patient as early neurosurgical intervention can both reduce the mortality rate and reduce the morbidity in these patients.

109.   What is not considered a factor behind the increased trauma death rate in rural areas?

a. Delayed time to reach a hospital

b. More severe injuries in rural hospitals

c. Poor EMS care in rural areas

d. Lack of trauma centers in rural areas

Answer: c. Even with excellent ATLS protocols and excellent EMS care, patients in rural areas have a higher rate of trauma-related deaths because of more serious injuries, delays in transport, and a lack of trauma centers in rural areas.

110.   The initial care of the patient with multiple traumatic injuries starts with what process?

a. Identification of where best to send the patient

b. Resuscitation of the patient

c. Thorough head-to-toe evaluation

d. Assessment of the most life-threatening injuries

Answer: d. The initial care of the multiple-trauma patient starts with a primary assessment of the most life-threatening injuries, shortly followed by resuscitation of the patient.

111.   In resuscitating a hemorrhaging patient, what is the volume expander of choice?

a. Lactated Ringer solution

b. Normal saline

c. D5W

d. Albumin solution

Answer: a. In initially managing hemorrhage, the solution of choice is lactated Ringer solution.

112.   What is the best way to get an assessment of the possibility of a spinal cord injury?

a. Evaluate the patient's level of consciousness

b. Do a brief sensory examination

c. Observe the patient's motor abilities

d. Assess the spinal column for edema or deformities

Answer: c. The best assessment of the patient's spinal cord status is to get an observation of their spontaneous motor abilities.

113.   You suspect the patient who is multiply-injured of having an impending brainstem herniation. What is not considered a treatment of choice for this?

a. IV mannitol

b. Cervical spine immobilization

c. Hyperventilation

d. Urgent neurosurgical consult

Answer: b. All of the above are good treatments for impending brainstem herniation except for cervical spine immobilization, which will not help the problem.

114.   Which is not considered an area assessed well by the FAST examination?

a. Brain

b. Pelvis

c. Pericardium

d. Abdomen

Answer: a. The FAST examination will assess the pelvis, the pericardium, the chest and the abdomen. The brain is not directly evaluated in this type of evaluation.

115.   The CT scan is sensitive in determining injuries to many body areas injured in a multiple trauma situation. What part of the body is least likely to be helped by doing a CT scan?

a. Brain

b. Cervical spine

c. Chest

d. Extremities

Answer: d. The CT scan is the definitive radiologic study, which can be done on most body areas where trauma is suspected. It is not as helpful in evaluating the patient's extremity injuries, however.

116.   What area of the body is best managed by doing strategic arterial embolization when arterial bleeding is suspected in the trauma patient?

a. Coronary arteries

b. Pelvic arteries

c. Cerebral arteries

d. Extremity arteries

Answer: b. The pelvis is an area where rapid angiographic embolization can be done faster than surgery to stop uncontrolled arterial bleeding.

117. What is the purpose of putting a 90-degree angle and the wrist twisting in the placement of sutures?

a. It allows for inversion of the skin layers.

b. It decreases the risk of infection.

c. It allows for eversion of the skin layers.

d. There is better approximation of the skin edges.

Answer: c. The purpose of using a 90-degree angle and twisting the wrist in laceration repair is to allow for better eversion of the skin layers, which is better for cosmesis in the final result.

118. What is the major reason why lacerations are generally repaired?

a. It reduces the risk of infection.

b. It helps achieve hemostasis

c. It improves function of the affected part.

d. All of the above are reasons to repair a laceration.

Answer: d. All of the reasons listed are good reasons to repair a laceration.

119. What is the main anesthetic used in children's facial wounds?

a. Topical lidocaine and prilocaine cream

b. 2 percent lidocaine and bicarbonate

c. 0.25 percent bupivacaine

d. 1 percent lidocaine

Answer: a. The main anesthetic used in children's facial wounds is EMLA, which is topical lidocaine and prilocaine cream.

120. The patient has a laceration of the face that needs repair. After how long can you not repair the wound because of an increase in infection rate?

a. 8 hours

b. 12 hours

c. 24 hours

d. 36 hours

Answer: c. A well-vascularized area such as the face can be treated with primary closure within 24 hours of the time of injury. Anything after that will result in an increase in infection.

121. How many tetanus shots does a person need, at a minimum, to be considered protected against Clostridium tetani?

a. Two

b. Three

c. Four

d. Five

Answer: b. It basically takes a minimum of three injections of tetanus to be considered protected against Clostridium tetani.

122.   About how many years should there be between tetanus booster shots?

a. Three

b. Five

c. Seven

d. Ten

Answer: d. A tetanus booster shot should be given every ten years to have tetanus protection.

123.   Which aspect of a patient's history is least likely to be helpful in evaluating a patient with a laceration?

a. Past surgical history

b. Tetanus status

c. Medical history for chronic diseases and immunodeficiency states

d. Allergies to Latex, tape, local anesthesia, and antibiotics

Answer: a. All of the above are important; however, the past surgical history is the least helpful aspect of the patient's historical information.

124.   A surgical consult should be obtained in all but the following situations?

a. Deep hand or foot lacerations

b. Severely contaminated wounds

c. Avulsion of the tip of the finger

d. Wound involving tendon, nerves, arteries, or bone

Answer: c. All of the above are good wounds for referring to a surgeon; however, wounds involving the tip of the finger cannot be repaired surgically, especially if they are small so a surgical consult is less likely to be an issue.

125.   Where should a staple technique not be used?

a. Scalp

b. Trunk

c. Arm

d. Face

Answer: d. Staples should be used on thicker skin where cosmesis is not as important. The skin on the face is not very thick and there will not be a good cosmetic result if staples are used.

126. The most severe psychiatric emergency the provider could encounter is what type of emergency?

a. A psychotic patient who hears voices telling him to harm the president of the United States

b. A patient who has taken an acetaminophen overdose but is still alive

c. A patient who is very depressed and thinking about purchasing a firearm

d. A manic patient who believes he can fly and wants to jump off a tall building

Answer: b. The most severe end of the spectrum involves the patient who has already perpetrated their aggressive act (such as having already taken an overdose) but has survived their attempt. These patients need psychiatric and medical attention.

127. What is the best predictor of suicidal completion in a patient who has suicidal ideation?

a. Having a previous suicidal act that was unsuccessful

b. Having a suicidal plan

c. Having feelings of hopelessness and despair

d. Having a recent life stressor

Answer: a. The best predictor of suicidal intent is a past history of suicidal actions that were previously unsuccessful.

128. Which patient is more likely to have a completed suicide?

a. A 10-year-old child whose parents have recently divorced.

b. A 19-year-old female who recently broke up with her boyfriend.

c. A 30-year-old male with an exacerbation of manic-depressive disease.

d. A 65-year-old male with a recent diagnosis of terminal cancer.

Answer: d. While suicidal ideation and suicidal attempts tend to occur at a higher rate among young people, older males, especially those with medical problems, have a higher risk for completing a suicide.

129. In evaluating a patient in the emergency department, what percentage of patients who have previously attempted suicide will have a completed suicide in the future?

a. Five percent

b. Ten percent

c. Twenty-five percent

d. Fifty percent

Answer: c. The lifetime prevalence of completed suicide in a patient who has previously attempted suicide is about 25 percent.

130.   Why might a blood and alcohol screen be important in evaluating a patient with a psychiatric emergency?

a. The patient may have already taken an overdose of illicit drugs or alcohol.

b. The intoxicated patient is not likely to be safe driving home from the hospital.

c. The intoxicated patient is less likely to have true meaning behind their intent.

d. The patient on drugs or alcohol has impaired judgment and is more likely to act on their intent.

Answer: d. The patient intoxicated on drugs or alcohol has an impairment of judgment and is more likely to act on their aggressive intent.

131.   What would a first-line medication be for the management of the aggressive psychotic patient?

a. Neuroleptic medication

b. Benzodiazepine medication

c. Mood stabilizer

d. Barbiturate medication

Answer: a. The best way to manage aggressive behavior in psychosis is to make use of neuroleptic medications. These will decrease delusions and hallucinations, and can improve the patient's risk for carrying out an aggressive intent.

132.   What type of toxicology test will best yield an accurate quantitative testing of the substance versus just a qualitative assessment?

a. Sputum

b. Saliva

c. Urine

d. Blood

Answer: d. Blood testing is about the only method of getting a good quantitative measurement of a given drug or toxic substance. Testing of the other areas of the body will only yield a qualitative measurement of the presence of the substance.

133.   The taking of certain cough medications can adversely affect the results of a test. What toxicology test substance might mistakenly return as positive?

a. Alcohol

b. Amphetamines

c. Cocaine

d. Marijuana

Answer: a. There can be a positive alcohol or opiate test when a patient takes a cough preparation so this must be noted when a patient receives a toxicology screening test.

134.   Saliva testing is a good method of determining drug use. How long does a drug remain measurable in the saliva after using it?

a. Eight hours

b. Twelve hours

c. One day

d. Three days

Answer: c. The use of a drug within 24 hours or 1 day will be detectable in a saliva test of most drugs of abuse.

135.   There are several drugs that cause encephalopathy by having an increased serum ammonia level. What drugs do not generally do this?

a. Acetaminophen

b. Cocaine

c. Carbon tetrachloride

d. Valproic acid

Answer: b. All of the above will cause an encephalopathy from elevated ammonia levels except for cocaine, which doesn't cause hepatic encephalopathy.

136.   Some drugs, when taken in excess or on a prolonged basis will lead to an ischemic or hemorrhagic stroke. Which drugs do not cause this phenomenon?

a. LSD

b. Cocaine

c. Amphetamines

d. Ephedrine

Answer: a. Cocaine, amphetamines, ephedrine, and phenylpropanolamine can all cause an ischemic or hemorrhagic stroke. LSD and dextromethorphan do not cause a stroke.

137.   There are several treatments that can be used for altered mental status patients, especially when the etiology is unknown. What is not included in these treatments?

a. Oxygen

b. Lactulose

c. Dextrose

d. Thiamine

Answer: b. Any of the above will help reverse the symptoms of altered mental status if the etiology is unknown except for lactulose, which is used for hepatic encephalopathy only.

138.   Which exposure in the system can lead to cardiac arrhythmias?

a. Mercury

b. Doxorubicin

c. Cocaine

d. Sildenafil

Answer: a. Both mercury and MDMA (Ecstasy) can cause cardiac arrhythmias. The others can cause heart problems but not cardiac arrhythmias.

139.   Which exposure has the potential to lead to a hypotensive episode?

a. Mercury

b. MDMA

c. Doxorubicin

d. Sildenafil

Answer: d. Sildenafil is an erectile dysfunction drug that can cause a hypotensive episode if taken along with nitrates.

140.   When it comes to ototoxic drugs, which drug do you least have to worry about?

a. Phenytoin

b. Gentamycin

c. Aspirin

d. Cisplatin

Answer: a. All of the drugs are considered to be ototoxic except for phenytoin, which generally does not result in any type of ototoxicity.

Printed in Great Britain
by Amazon

79429432R00099